Understanding Self-Worth

Understanding Self-Worth: A Guide to Worth-Conscious Theory and Psychotherapeutic Practice is a guide for psychotherapists confounded by the struggle of working with clients who present with a pervasive pattern of denied self-worth.

When self-worth is perceived as conditional or denied altogether, clients may become complicit in creating a lost-worth story—the story they tell that keeps them denying their own worth. The denial may include generational abusive and/or intrusive injunctions that go against their lived truth.

Psychotherapists will come away from this book with a deep understanding of the importance of attending to the degree of trauma experienced when the client's self-worth is separated from their individual truth. Moreover, where there is worth-based trauma, the psychotherapist will learn models both for helping clients gently and honestly reestablish a worthy and true sense of self and for consciously guiding clients toward recovery of human worth as a birthright.

Dawna Daigneault, EdS, LPC, CCTP, is a writer, speaker, and professional counselor with twenty years of experience. She specializes in serving clients with self-worth challenges that complicate client trauma.

Chris Brown, MS, PhD, is professor emerita in the Psychology and Counseling Department at the University of Missouri–Kansas City. She is a licensed psychologist with more than forty years of experience providing psychotherapy to culturally diverse populations.

Understanding Self-Worth

A Guide to Worth-Conscious Theory and Psychotherapeutic Practice

Dawna Daigneault and Chris Brown

Routledge
Taylor & Francis Group

NEW YORK AND LONDON

Designed cover image: Shutterstock

First published 2026
by Routledge
605 Third Avenue, New York, NY 10158

and by Routledge
4 Park Square, Milton Park, Abingdon, Oxon, OX14 4RN

ISBN: 978-1-032-98638-8 (hbk)
ISBN: 978-1-032-98634-0 (pbk)
ISBN: 978-1-003-59973-9 (ebk)

DOI: 10.4324/9781003599739

Typeset in Adobe Caslon Pro
by SPi Technologies India Pvt Ltd (Straive)

This book is dedicated to my courageous and compassionate sons, conscientious husband, and kindhearted stepdaughters. I am grateful for all my friends and family who've made honoring self-worth a mutual joy. One wish I have, as I share my little model, is for everyone who reads this book to learn something new and beneficial about their self-worth that they can continue sharing. ~**Dawna Daigneault**

To every reader who has ever doubted their self-worth and to those who have found their purpose in helping others restore their self-worth, may the words in this book provide the strength to live your truth, the power to love yourself unconditionally, and the courage to pursue a journey of growth and healing all while knowing you are worthy. Finally, to my dear family and friends, this book is also for you. You inspire me simply by being who you are. ~**Chris Brown**

CONTENTS

ILLUSTRATIONS

Figures

Tables

PREFACE

An esteemed emperor wanted to renovate a sacred temple and issued a decree throughout the city inviting anyone who wanted a chance to work on the project. This ancient Taoist story (Lin, 2010) focused on the craftspeople the emperor hoped to employ in the renovation. Many groups of workers responded to the emperor's invitation. However, only two groups impressed the emperor enough to be allowed to proceed with restoring the temple. Because the nature of this project was of great worth in the community, the two groups were issued a trial phase, which involved completing a smaller project/temple first. The two groups had differing ideas about what would enhance the beauty of the temple. The first group of artisans had been doing projects in the city for decades; they had impressive skills and experience with design. The second group consisted of monks dedicated to returning the temple to its former glory; they were committed to its restoration.

Two smaller temples were chosen, and one was assigned to each group to prove to the emperor which improvement plan for the sacred temple would be appropriate to the task's significance. The groups were escorted to the smaller temples and given all the supplies needed to finish their work. They worked on the two smaller buildings according to their ideas of beauty. On the last day, the emperor returned to judge the finished project.

The artisans' building looked brand new. They had skillfully repainted all the walls and roof with bright and commanding colors. The emperor, accompanied by his ministers, were all impressed by the sight and praised the artists. Next, they visited the building the monks had renovated. As he and his ministers approached the second building, they did not see new paint on the exterior. This was not very reassuring. When they arrived at the old building, they realized it was spotless and polished to its original beauty. The monks had meticulously cleaned every surface, restored the structures, and revealed the details of the venerable artistry. Its ancient style and character were reclaimed and preserved. The emperor felt a sense of awe.

The emperor and his ministers discussed the difference between the two buildings. The efforts of the monks brought beauty out of the building, as though they had brought it back to life. The artisans had covered all the original beauty with paint, which, while attractive, would fade. The difference to the emperor was stark; he preferred how the monks accepted and revered the sacred place. They had honored its serenity rather than demanding attention with new colorful painting that covered up the temple. He gave the final project to the monks because they had understood the worth of the place they would restore.

The story of the emperor and the temple can be personally meaningful when readers recognize the symbolism embedded in the details. The temple is the self, and the group of artisans used their skill to cover up the self to make it appear new and improved. The Taoist conceptualization of how the artisans approached the task was that they desired to be impressive and to win recognition. The emperor represented wisdom and power, and he understood that the artisans' use of pretty paint was the art of concealment, which covered up underlying issues rather than recognizing the repairs needed. The Taoist conceptualization of how the monks approached the task was that they focused on their understanding of the internal essence of the space, which allowed them to remove the accumulated dirt and thereby see what repairs were essential. The monks aimed to remove anything that obscured the temple's original nature, symbolically representing every human being's true essence. In other words, they desired to discover what was hidden and to reveal what was real.

This story allows us, in modern-day mental health, to consider two different ways in which people deal with something that seems to have lost its worth. As a person, we can cover up what seems unworthy or allow it to be obscured; in doing so, however, what is covered remains more accurate than the paint on top. A duality can exist where worth exists but is not honored or even recognized as essential to the person. That can be disconcerting for the person, shifting one's mental state toward continual self-consciousness about what is hidden, why it is being hidden, and how much more hiding is required to be acceptable.

The journey to understanding self-worth can feel like an arduous task. Self-worth is the reality that our existence matters (it does not need to be earned) and that we are valued enough to continue the journey to becoming ourselves. It is easy to get lost in the noise of expectations that are held by families and larger systems that have obscured our worth. Furthermore, we may feel the need to cover up aspects of ourselves that others deem unworthy, thereby curating versions of ourselves that reject our uniqueness and/or differences.

Worth-conscious theory focuses on self-worth as being original to human nature. As psychotherapists, we can look for ways to brush away cobwebs and wipe away any debris that has accumulated over the years obscuring a client's view of their self-worth as a birthright. We view all human worth that has been painted over as something that is still there waiting to be remembered. We can also be aware of the layers of paint that others have applied in the family system to *improve* how the family is perceived in their community by altering how a member can (or cannot) present themselves. The alteration conveys that worth is conditional and that some individual truths should not be seen. Painting over undesirable qualities can be required in some systems; it can be taught in some families as an unspoken requirement for acceptance. A member of a conditional-worth-oriented system can become a client in psychotherapy. A client with denied self-worth from systemic conditions can learn to keep a fresh coat of paint applied to gain approval without understanding they are losing sight of their self-worth as it becomes buried under layers.

Our book is born out of our passion for helping individuals recognize their self-worth as a birthright. Each chapter is designed to assist psychotherapists with understanding self-worth and worth-conscious theory, while providing practical tools and strategies to strengthen their client's innate capacity to be true to self and self-worth. Specifically, in our book, we attend to the struggle between having a worth-conscious or self-conscious frame of reference. They are considered opposing concepts because one promotes wellness, whereas the other demotes it. Like the story of the artisans and the temple, a client experiencing denied self-worth may be unaware of how they perpetuate a systemic requirement that alters or covers up something original and significant. We invite psychotherapists who are working with clients that have endured denial of their self-worth to glean the client's story about having their self-worth affirmed or not. They can listen to and learn what the client knows about themselves (truth and worth) and their attempts (by others or themselves) to make-over or restore their worth to their truth. In the parable of the temple, the client is the forgotten building. However, they can also be co-builders with the psychotherapist, bringing knowledge and skills to the process. In addition, the client can become the wise emperor in their own story by observing, learning, and making informed decisions about what reveals their original nature (worth and truth) and how to reclaim it.

We endeavor to explore and explain how worth-based consciousness contributes to an overall sense of well-being, and how self-consciousness, although common in some systems, is often angst-ridden. Those feelings of angst (such as, am I worthy, or is my truth worth seeing and restoring) can develop into a severe level of fear-based anxiety if the client is afraid that their worth and truth will never be enough. Self-conscious anxiety can become severe and runs the risk of becoming pathological, manifesting as insecurities, over-striving, comparison-driven anger, hopelessness, and so forth. Throughout our book, we seek to foster an understanding of the unrelenting symptoms often at the root of a learned pattern of denied self-worth, which will be important in recovering self-worth through a healing journey which includes listening, learning, understanding, and developing worth-based consciousness. Our primary audience, psychotherapists, will be introduced to the importance of recognizing a pattern of denied self-worth in their clients and the degree of impaired well-being experienced by the client. In subsequent chapters, multiple factors such as components of our model, unique client circumstances, and systemic causes are presented to assist professionals in identifying, addressing, and alleviating their client's worth-denying thoughts, feelings, and actions. Our book offers a solid understanding of self-worth as an essential component of the human story, and that honoring self-worth is a work of restoration.

In the pages that follow, you will encounter examples of triumph and struggle, and exercises to help clients understand and affirm their self-worth. Our hope is that psychotherapists who are confounded by the struggle of working with clients who present with a pervasive pattern of denied self-worth will find our book a valuable resource for helping their clients to gently and honestly reestablish a worthy and true sense of self.

Reference

Lin, D. (2010). *The Tao of success: The five ancient rings of destiny.* Tarcher/Penguin.

INTRODUCTION

Self-worth, often used interchangeably with self-esteem, is a critical component of psychological health. Whereas self-worth influences how individuals perceive themselves, interact with others, and approach life's challenges, self-esteem refers to what one thinks, feels and believes about themselves. More importantly, self-worth fosters a deep understanding of one's value and unique significance. The professional community of psychotherapists and mental health professionals has extensively explored the implications of self-worth on overall well-being for decades. We argue that self-worth is an inherent birthright bestowed to everyone. Similarly, advocates of self-worth assert that basic worth and equal moral worth are based on facts about what contributes to or threatens wellness and a flourishing life (Sangiovanni, 2023). In *Understanding Self-Worth: A Guide to Worth-Conscious Theory and Psychotherapeutic Practice*, we look to the inherent nature of self-worth as universal and as being significant in understanding human dignity. We want our readers to understand that self-worth is a birthright that can be developed and realized over a lifetime as a form of actualization.

Understanding Self-Worth: A Guide to Worth-Conscious Theory and Psychotherapeutic Practice promotes well-being as a therapeutic objective and provides psychotherapists with a framework that addresses clients' denial of self-worth. An important aim of our book is to introduce readers to worth-conscious theory (WCT), which supports clients' overall well-being by helping them meet their self-worth needs. We offer insight into how WCT was constructed and why specific psychology and philosophy concepts were used both as foundational to the theory and as scaffolding to give formation to this novel way of looking at self-worth. One of the main differences in WCT as compared to theories which lump self-worth and self-esteem together as the same idea is that self-worth is solid and does not fluctuate; it does not rise and fall like self-esteem. We promote that all human beings have worth that is unconditional, intrinsic, and absolute (Sangiovanni, 2023) and that the solid nature of worth enhances the human experience by encouraging us toward worth-based well-being. Two main components of WCT are personal truth (i.e., what we know about ourselves) and self-worth (i.e., how we honor who we are), which can be congruent throughout life and thereby contribute to well-being. The truth that one person experiences about self may differ from what is true for another person, and this may be best understood through having self-worth needs met (or not) during the early developmental years.

Affirmed self-worth, sometimes referred to as high self-worth, is associated with positive outcomes such as resilience, happiness, and effective coping strategies (Rogers, 1961). In *Understanding Self-Worth: A Guide to Worth-Conscious Theory and Psychotherapeutic Practice*, we tie self-worth to having a birthright (i.e., birthright self-worth [BSW]), which endows every person with a vital frame of reference that can enhance life satisfaction and benefit mental health (Seligman, 2011). In our book, we explore the connection between affirmed self-worth and wellness by describing the values associated with well-being. The seven WCT wellness values that are embodied in BSW (i.e., wholeness, justice, goodness, uniqueness, truth, self-sufficiency, meaningfulness) are integral to the application of the theory. Within the WCT framework, self-worth is key in developing individuality. First, WCT affirms that every infant has BSW (i.e., a foundational privilege to just be), which includes being supported in their self-discovery of self-worth needs and life needs. Second, WCT encourages the embodiment of BSW as a self-supporting life philosophy. There are many complimentary concepts within WCT described in depth in the book, including:

- What a lifelong pattern of realized self-worth is.
- How to recognize and rewrite a lost-worth story.
- What systemic exigencies are and how they exist in families.
- Which worth-denying habits (injunctions, conditions, or counterfeits) affect BSW.
- How inherent and acquired values can cause confusion.
- When competing values become problematic to a solid sense of self.

We hope that reading our book will provide insight into self-worth as a vital aspect of the healing process and that psychotherapists will learn how to recognize a pattern of denied self-worth in their clients. Understanding the unrelenting symptoms that may be at the root of denied self-worth begins the healing journey. In other words, when a lost-worth story (LWS) is present, the WCT approach encourages the psychotherapist to support their client as they share their LWS without fearing that their story will become even more true. In the WCT approach, psychotherapists are introduced to tools that they can give to their clients to help them address their destructive habit of living from a lost-worth narrative while also deconstructing their LWS, and learning to utilize building blocks that will help them to construct a self-worth-based life script.

Disclaimer

This guidebook is written by licensed clinical psychotherapists for licensed professionals in the mental health field to use with their clients. Although self-help enthusiasts can benefit from reading the material, we strongly recommend that professional counseling be sought if notable reactions are experienced (e.g., difficulty sleeping, feeling triggered, intense sadness, or racing thoughts) due to a personal connection with the content in this book, including the stories and examples that are offered to assist with the application of the theoretical framework. The stories and examples used in the book represent our work with clients and interactions with others over the years. In addition to the use of pseudonyms, personal details have been altered to ensure anonymity and to protect the identities of others. In some instances, permission has been granted to use the story.

References

Rogers, C. R. (1961). *On becoming a person: A therapist's view of psychotherapy.* Boston, MA: Houghton Mifflin.

Sangiovanni, A. (2023). Are we of equal moral worth?

Seligman, M. E. (2011). *Flourish: A visionary new understanding of happiness and wellness.* New York: Free Press.

1

THEORETICAL FRAMEWORK

Well-being can be cultivated through various means, including engaging in individual and relational processes that seek to enhance self-worth. Martin Seligman (2013) provided a definition of well-being that includes one's thoughts, feelings, and capacity for engagement in healthy relationships with others. In essence, well-being is a combination of positive emotions, engagement, meaning, relationships and accomplishment (p. 25). Attaining well-being may be a desired outcome for many clients when they turn to psychotherapy for help. *Understanding Self-Worth: A Guide to Worth-Conscious Theory and Psychotherapeutic Practice* promotes well-being as a therapeutic objective and provides psychotherapists with a framework that addresses client self-worth denial in an effort to support their overall well-being through helping them meet self-worth needs. Within the worth-conscious theory (WCT) framework, the inclusion of both subjective and objective variables that affect personal worth, and therefore impact well-being, is recognized as significant to enjoying a healthy human experience. The subjective variables include how the individual's thoughts and feelings about having self-worth denied or affirmed inform their sense of well-being. The objective variables include how the system the individual was raised (or currently lives) in supports self-worth as a birthright (a fact) or supports conditions which deny that birthright and how that can also inform well-being.

DOI: 10.4324/9781003599739-1

A significant element of *Understanding Self-Worth: A Guide to Worth Conscious Theory and Psychotherapeutic Practice* is that human beings have birthright self-worth (BSW), which includes the capacity to dignify individual personhood (thoughts and feelings) through affirming BSW in self and others (action/engagement), and through increased awareness and consideration of the worth of individuals (accomplishment). In essence, becoming worth-conscious can be a lifelong wellness practice. Within our theoretical model, well-being is both subjective and objective and includes the possession and consistent affirmation of BSW that is critical to building the four pillars of self-worth. The four pillars of self-worth are being self-aware, and possessing self-respect, self-esteem, and self-confidence and are instrumental in understanding individuals' life challenges, presenting issues, and learning how to assist individuals in repairing and maintaining their worth. In our book, we describe a journey from birth through adulthood in the course of which a person can become aware and develop their innate capacity to be true to self and self-worth, thereby diminishing the psychological pain that develops in the absence of congruency between self and self-worth.

WCT consists of a set of philosophical and psychological constructs that will inform and enhance well-being through understanding and supporting BSW and assisting clients to realize their self-worth even when it has been denied.

WCT is a theoretical model with philosophical underpinnings such as:

1. Meaning and eventual fulfillment in life is related to understanding the role of self-worth in society and within self as an individual.
2. Human suffering is magnified by denial of self-worth relationally and independently.
3. Liberation from conditions which include abusive and intrusive injunctions (i.e., direct statements and attributions about 'what the child is' which are potent parental instructions) is essential to personal realization of self-worth.

WCT proposes a framework that addresses the early exposure to relational rules/requirements that deny self-worth of members within a system, and the later development of the four pillars of self-worth to reaffirm the dignified birthright of self-worth and the ability to have realized self-worth (RSW) despite the early practice of denial within the family or larger system. RSW is the ability, knowledge, and consistent effort to actualize a lifelong pattern of affirming self-worth.

The multifaceted three-component practice shared by the Dalai Lama (Kabat-Zinn & Davidson, 2011) to achieve dharma (the alleviation of suffering through overcoming the inner causes of suffering) is similar to the process that started to unfold in the development of WCT. The three components in achieving dharma include, first, having a theory or worldview. Our worth-conscious theoretical model directs the psychotherapist to look at the outer and inner world of the client, including learning if they have a self-conscious or worth-conscious frame of reference. The second component of achieving dharma is meditation, which is the practice of transforming the mind and investigating how the mind experiences and comprehends itself and the world. WCT supports a process similar to meditation in that a purposeful worth-conscious-producing practice is emphasized and includes an investigation of self as worthy, and also insight into why a client is or is not conscious of their individual worth, which supports being mindful of their worthiness. The third component is conduct or action, which supports cultivation of heart and mind. Our WCT framework invites psychotherapists to assist clients in looking at the development of self over their lifetime and how worth was affirmed or denied in childhood in their family system. Following this review of the development of self across the lifespan, clients are invited to address how they have affirmed or denied BSW. An important goal is for clients to understand that when worth-affirming practices were in place in their family system or are presently co-created in psychotherapy, they are well-positioned to experience an enduring practice of worth-consciousness that supports well-being.

Three additional components of the WCT framework are:

1. *Point of View.* Human worth is a birthright that can be affirmed or denied.
2. *Investigation and Insight.* The attainment of knowledge about self-worth and how it is affirmed or denied is possible even within systems where the rules about denying self-worth are rigid (exigencies). Insight can be gained about personal self-worth and

new practices to affirm self-worth can begin without permission from others in the system.

3. *Development and Realization.* How we conduct ourselves can affirm self-worth. Because BSW is endowed on every human, anyone can access it within themselves, and then develop a solid sense of self-worth. Development of the four pillars of self-worth is more challenging when an individual lives in a system that denies their BSW. Even though affirming BSW can be difficult within a denial-based system, those difficulties do not preclude someone from realizing their self-worth through patience and practice, over their own lifetime.

WCT aligns with aspects of postmodern philosophy. Some of the postmodern ideology that fits include that diversity is valued, individual experience is identified as important, personal meaning is possible, and truth is not independent of context. Postmodern thinkers' question and explore what has come to be a social norm in order to deconstruct a tradition that may no longer serve the greater good (Foster, 1983). The term conscious in WCT was chosen to refer to the ability that individuals have to become aware of self and self-worth or to be conscious of self and self-worth as inalienable. This may be an innate knowing that helps humans align with their BSW and can cause mental/emotional pain when a person is not allowed to be true to themselves and stay aligned with their BSW.

WCT incorporates ideology from interpersonal neurobiology (IPNB), including the idea that humans share a common genetic inheritance and long for warm attachment with trustworthy family and friends (Badenoch, 2023). This longing speaks to the significance of recognizing and honoring a common human need such as self-worth, which starts early in life. IPNB trainer Bonnie Badenoch (2023) shared that IPNB is a scientifically based, interdisciplinary study of how humans influence one another's neural landscape from moment to moment. In these moments, self-worth can be affirmed or denied, and the denial can become a pattern of misinterpretation of a person's truth and/or worth. In other words, the pattern that is learned in the system can be accepted and internalized by the client whether it is an accurate or inaccurate portrayal of the client's truth and or worth.

The mental experience of our nervous system continuously searching for a true presence with others, which provides a type of safety was promoted by Porges (2011). To continuously search for a true and safe presence with others illustrates how crucial it is that we experience our self-worth and personal truth as safe in the presence of others. A trustworthy and sustained interpersonal connection can provide a safe haven during the developmental phase of life. This safe haven allows one to gain perspective about what is true for them as an individual over time while also remaining worthy through the experience.

Influential Theories

Narrative Therapy

One of the early influences on the development of WCT as its own model was narrative therapy. Narrative therapy emerged from systemic family therapy and was seen as a post-modern social constructionism therapy (i.e., knowledge, meaning, and identity are constructed through interaction with others; Anderson, 2003). Social constructionism therapy is concerned with how meaning as a social construct can create social change. Sociologists Berger and Luckmann (1967) developed the theory of social construction of reality, which promoted the idea that repeated action can become a pattern that it is more economical to repeat. Humans can create and sustain new phenomena (patterns) through communal practice (Vera, 2016). Parents who *externalize* their thoughts/feelings on the world, such as sharing a story which includes ideas about being worthy or unworthy can set up a thinking process which can become a pattern for their child. As the parent's story is shared, the ideas become an *object* of consciousness for listeners, such as children, who may accept the story content as fact. If the ideas in the story become a fact (objective truth), they can then become pervasive and *internalized* in the consciousness of larger systems (i.e., family or community). This process results in the next generation taking for granted that the contents of the story are facts or truths (Burr, 2015).

Narrative therapy recognizes that a client's life is storied, and that narrative is an organizing principle for action (Sarbin, 1986). Psychotherapists using narrative as a modality recognize the importance of the relational process and the highly personal aspect of a client's interpretation of life events (Larner, 2004). Michael White and David Epston (1990) developed a therapeutic approach while working with families that focused on how each member of the family has a personal narrative that helped them organize their life and make coherent meaning from experiences within their family system and culture (Murdock, 2004). A dominant narrative can be created and believed by a client even when certain aspects of their lived experience do not support that particular story. For example, although a female client may have successfully competed against men in chess, she may still believe that women are inferior. In other words, there is a negative characterization that dominates the sense of self regardless of the positive attributes that are being experienced (White & Epston, 1990). Foucault (1979) and Foucault and Colin (1980) remind us that a dominant narrative has power to construct norms from ideas that are given a truth status thereby normalizing their use from generation to generation. Some universal truths that society has adhered to came from modernism, which is a cultural construct based on specific conditions, and therefore limited in its usefulness to future generations (Foster, 1983). When sitting with a client who started talking about feeling worthless, a specific story emerged. A separate but uniquely personal story about a loss that hurt more deeply than other offenses the client had endured was shared. The sharing of the loss made the client cry, which was accompanied by feeling worthless and with a big dose of individual shame. The first author's earliest experiences as a psychotherapist with clients who shifted into a shame-based personal narrative included learning a lesson about how to follow the client into the most unfriendly space within them—space that they kept hidden from the eyes of others. I learned to recognize the existence of a story about lost worth that was held by the client in an internal mental/emotional space they did not want to visit. The importance of being invited by the client to enter into this space with them was an honor. I gained understanding that to return the honor of the invitation with a type of reverence was helpful. Reverence is simply the highest form of respect, so I let the client set the pace as we proceeded together into their story.

The Role of Shame and Denied Self-Worth. It is important for psychotherapists to recognize when shame causes their client to rapidly shift away from positive to negative affect in an autopilot transition to parasympathetic override (i.e., dominance) without their full awareness (Cozolino, 2010). The shift from a positive to a negative affective state can occur as a result of clients having expected a positive reaction from caregivers or important others only to receive a negative response/emotion. Parasympathetic dominance can be indicated by the presence of symptoms that contribute to lethargy, low motivation, and depression. This state of parasympathetic override is not the place to continue WCT; instead the use of trauma-informed care protocols is recommended (see Chapter 5).

The negative impact of shame should not be minimized. However, shame is normal, not pathological. It is how we handle shame that makes it maladaptive (Lewis, 1992). More precisely, maladaptive responses to shame can include various coping mechanisms such as *avoidance* (i.e., withdraw socially or failure to confront one's feelings, which can lead to isolation and intensified feelings of shame), *anger* (i.e., inward: self-hatred, self-criticism; outward: hostility towards others), *perfectionism* (i.e., set unrealistic standards in an attempt to avoid the feelings of shame associated with failure or imperfection), and *substance abuse or self-destructive behaviors* (i.e., attempt to numb or escape the painful feelings associated with shame by consuming drugs/alcohol or engaging in self-destructive behaviors) to name a few. Whereas maladaptive styles of coping with shame can undermine interpersonal relationships and negatively impact emotional well-being, Lewis (1992) reminded us that shame is the self-conscious emotion that we negotiate most of our psychic lives, which is in opposition to being worth-conscious. He further noted that shame allows us to escape the painful gaze of others by collapsing into ourselves and withdrawing from threatening interactions. In addition to how we experience and handle shame, it is important to point out that shame is held in the body as a dysphoric affect, which includes a sense of humiliation, the collapse of positive self-view, a rupture in the continuity of self, and isolation marked by being cut off from one's surroundings while being viewed critically by others (Akhtar, 2016).

Of further import, shame can become a mechanism of social control when a child's positive interactions with a caregiver during the early months of their life are replaced in the second year of life with disapproval and anger (Cozolino, 2010). Moreover, Cozolino asserted that being able to successfully move from a state of shame to attunement (i.e., feeling close and connected to others) supports affect regulation (i.e., ability to control our emotional states) and contributes to the development of self-regulation (i.e., understanding and monitoring our thoughts, feelings, and behaviors and our reactions to situations around us). In WCT, we want clients to be able to self-regulate at a basic level so that they can become aware of their pattern of denied self-worth.

The shame-based story shared in the example above, and which many more clients have shared in therapy sessions, was eventually given a name. The name, lost-worth story (LSW), resonated with the first few clients I used it with because it aligned with what those clients believed had happened. They felt worthless in childhood because someone in their family system consistently denied their self-worth. This denial can include neglecting to affirm self-worth but most often the reference that was made to childhood and the sense that self-worth was lost somewhere, somehow was about words, judgments, or labels an adult used against them.

In narrative therapy the psychotherapist looks for *the telling* of the family story. In WCT, the psychotherapist is listening for the client's retelling of a LWS that seems to embed the denial of self-worth in their actions as a common part of everyday life. Retelling versions of the LWS to themselves may reinforce a patten of denying self-worth and allow that story to dominate. The client can perpetuate the negative impact that the LWS has on their life by adding new people to the outdated story, and reinforcing its meaning, even when that increases feelings of unworthiness. WCT psychotherapists will listen for the power that the LWS has over the client when it is retold and believed anew. From there, the client is helped to become more aware of the building blocks that are used in the story that are built on a foundation of conditions to BSW and therefore deny their self-worth.

In the WCT model, the negative impact on self-worth comes from actions and behaviors that deny self-worth, such as conditions placed on worthiness that are required for acceptance, counterfeits set up as desirable goals that replace realizing self-worth, injunctions (both abusive and intrusive), and social norms that allow for discrimination. Moreover, further negative impact on self-worth is experienced by verbal and emotional abuse, which are invisible; they do not leave a mark, so the negative impact felt is not always seen after the harm is done. How it is felt and where it lands is not completely understood, but it seems like self-worth can be negatively affected.

We acknowledge that the LWS may be older than the client. Some aspects of the LWS may have started generations before the client was born. "What if your client is not the original author of that story?" The WCT-trained psychotherapist may ask the client, "Could someone in your family have written parts of that story before it was shared with you?" When this question is asked, the psychotherapist will wait to see if the client is already aware of who may have contributed to this worth-denying story. If the client can easily connect their LWS to other family members' comments, experiences, or history, the psychotherapist lets the client continue to connect the dots. This effort to follow the client into their story and allow them to find a point of origin that existed before they did can be helpful in creating awareness of systemic norms that make room for stories that diminish self-worth in some or all the members. If a client is unable to connect their LWS to any past family member or event, the client and psychotherapist allow for the possibility that a point of origin exists, but may not need to be known in order to attend to the contents of the story that include denied self-worth.

Person-Centered Therapy

The person-centered approach is considered a humanistic theory, but it can also be recognized as a branch of the existential perspective. Carl Rogers was instrumental in championing a nondirective approach with clients which assumed that people are essentially trustworthy with great potential for self-understanding (Corey, 1991). According to Rogers (1980):

> It is that the individual has within himself or herself vast resources for self-understanding, for altering his or her self-concept, attitudes and self-directed behavior—and that these resources can be tapped if only a definable climate of facilitative psychological attitudes can be provided.
>
> (p. 115)

We appreciate the clarity of Rogers (1961) to recognize the importance of self-concept and resourcefulness of clients. The WCT-trained psychotherapist regards BSW and the ability to realize self-worth as one of the most important resources an individual is born with. Within the WCT framework, a client can learn to understand how their denied self-worth can impair self-concept and affirmed self-worth can strengthen self-concept. In psychotherapy, client and clinician work together to add worth-based attitudes and actions that solidify BSW to the client's worth-affirming routine of building the four pillars of worth to increase client well-being, as an individual, and hopefully positively impact the larger system too. We will show the ways that a psychotherapist can facilitate improved self-worth practices with a client in a safe climate through using self-awareness and mutual respect building blocks early in the counseling process to begin co-constructing four pillars of self-worth.

From the system where clients were raised, they bring a preformed pattern for how things were built (e.g., imitation pillars rather than pillars of worth) into their psychotherapy sessions. The preformed pattern shows up as statements clients make about conditions in their family or family of origin that must be followed or counterfeits to their BSW that they are expected to pursue, but do not feel true to self when engaged in those required pursuits. Building imitation pillars that are familiar in their family but fail to embolden their self-worth provides clients skills in building pillars, but not in building pillars that affirm their self-worth. In our WCT framework, if denied self-worth is the basis of building a sense of self (i.e., pillars of behavior made of life's moments) then the preformed structure may be built on conditions that become rigid rules that the person follows. Rogers (1961) referred to this preformed structure phenomenon as tightly held evaluations that cannot be relinquished easily. In fact, clients will even cram and twist their new experiences to fit the old requirements and continue to pigeonhole themselves with antiquated systemic rules. Clients who continue to believe that denying BSW is acceptable may recreate similar interactions with people who also use conditions of worth.

Rogers (1961) provided insight into aspects of the self that involve conditions of worth and unconditional worth. Both of those concepts have been borrowed to use in the primary model of WCT. The more conditions, and the severity of those conditions, that are placed on an individual's BSW, the less likely the client is to construct the four pillars of self-worth and therefore are less likely to experience RSW. Rogers described the maladjustment of self-concept a child can develop while in a system where the inner experience of self does not match up to the conditions placed on their worth in their family of origin. Conditions of worth (i.e., requirements for acceptance) are placed on the child instead of "love without conditions" (Gelso & Fretz, 1992, p. 272). Moreover, Rogers asserted that a climate of safety is essential for the client to feel worthy enough to be themself without trying to preserve the façade of a worthy self. To establish psychological safety in the therapeutic realm, the psychotherapist can accept the client with unconditional worth in their own right and irrespective of their present condition or behavior.

Maslow's Hierarchy of Needs

Maslow (1968) understood that the higher non-material needs are also basic needs. He included a long list of these higher basic needs, such as protection, safety, security, belonging, community, friendship, affection, love, respect, esteem, approval, dignity, self-respect, and "freedom for the fullest development of one's talents and capacities, actualization of the self" (p. 200). It is apparent from the basic needs listed above that Maslow was interested in what makes a human being better. In reviewing Maslow's hierarchy of needs (see Figure 1.1), we acknowledge the importance of each need that Maslow included and further believe that additional human needs exist in the first year of life. We assert that the upper-level needs of self-esteem and love and belonging are included as self-worth needs (i.e., intrinsic to each of the four pillars of self-worth) that should be relocated to the bottom of the structure. This move grants those two self-worth needs an important and earlier start as they are as vital as life needs in the first year of life. Keeping self-actualization at the top of the model but renaming it as realized self-worth, acknowledged the movement from becoming more conscious of the needed congruency between truth and worth to being worthy as a way of life. This restructuring created a visually altered hierarchical pyramid with a design that shows the progress a person can make from birthright self-worth through realizing self-worth in adulthood. The WCT pyramid, a reimagining of Maslow's hierarchy, shows that life needs, and self-worth needs can both begin to be fulfilled in the first year of life (see Figure 1.2).

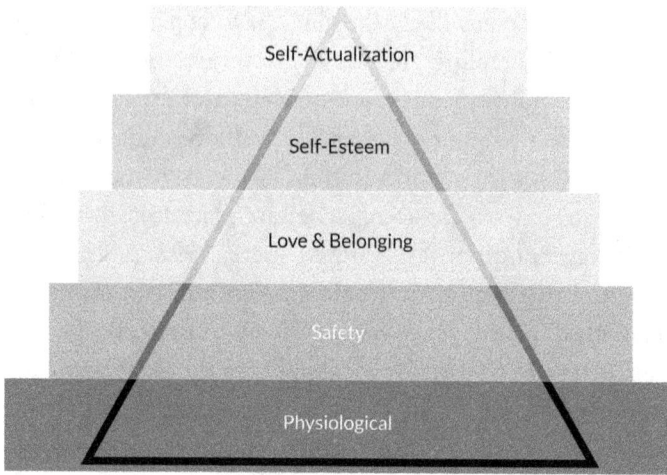

Figure 1.1 Maslow's Hierarchy of Needs.

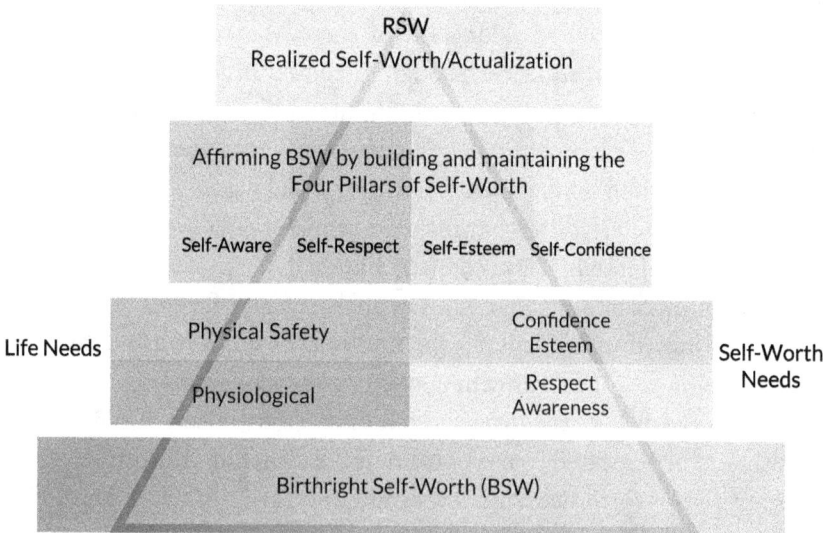

Figure 1.2 Worth-Conscious Theory Pyramid.

A final version of the WCT pyramid shows that when life needs and self-worth needs are met early in childhood, individuals are afforded a foundation of affirmed worth based on their authentic selves and are likely to have their BSW affirmed consistently in their family system. This consistent affirmation of BSW, allows individuals to become adept at affirming their own self-worth needs and build the four pillars of self-worth. They can continue to share worth-affirming building blocks within the family system and within new systems they encounter, while they build and eventually maintain the four pillars of self-worth throughout life and enjoy the well-being that comes from RSW.

Existential Theory and Therapy

Viktor Frankl (1992) described for millions of readers what it was like to be dehumanized. As a doctor of neurology and psychiatry, he was well trained to observe and understand human nature. He used that training to pay attention to himself and the other inmates being held captive at a concentration camp during WWII. Frankl was dedicated to keeping his humanity in the midst of a system that was deconstructing the mind, body, and soul of WWII prisoners. He shared the steps that he saw people go through as they slowly surrendered to their fate (loss of dignity and a sense of insignificance). The painful and disempowering three-step process can become a reality for the most unfortunate people in history. As described by Frankl in *Man's Search for Meaning*, the three stages occur when someone is devalued within a system where their worth is ignored by others and where the existence of dignity is only denied to some.

Step 1, shock about the undignified situation sets in. Disbelief is a normal reaction to the worth-denying actions of others. If the situation does not return to normal (BSW is recognized again), then the erosion of self as unvalued continues.

Step 2, apathy increases. Not wanting to feel the degradation of being unworthy to others is a defense mechanism. Apathy makes things easier at first, but can evolve into an emotional death. People can surrender to a worth-denying narrative (LWS) created by others and eventually make it their own personal narrative too.

Step 3, personal values are surrendered. Frankl asserted that when a prisoner stopped struggling to save their self-respect, surrender of their last inner freedom would occur. Non-being took over and human beings with their own minds ceased to be. Losing the will to value ourselves as deserving basic human dignity requires the surrender of a belief in BSW. Routine denial of human worth during WWII became the last personal surrender of many hopeless hearts.

According to Frankl (1992) and cited in Daigneault and Brown (2023), the will-to-meaning is a primary motivational force in every human being and therefore essential to healthy psychological functioning. Frankl posited that the conscious striving for meaning in life results in a dimension of human existence whereby an individual experiences values and true morality. However, when life situations frustrate the will-to-meaning, making it difficult or impossible to discover meaning in life, the individual experiences what Frankl distinctively refers to as an existential vacuum. The existential vacuum results in the individual experiencing a permeating sense of boredom and apathy in life, which leads to an aimless existence. We draw from Frankl's work by asserting that having self-worth is a birthright and being worth-conscious promotes genuine meaning in life.

WCT borrows from existential therapy in that it shares some of the dimensions of the human condition as they relate to self-worth or a sense of having BSW. The basic set of existential therapy dimensions outline important aspects of understanding deep human experiences (Corey, 1991). Corey provided a simple format of the dimensions of the human condition:

1. The Capacity for Self-Awareness
2. Freedom and Responsibility
3. Striving for Identity and Relationship to Others
   a. The courage to be.
   b. The experience of aloneness.
   c. The experience of relatedness.

4. The Search for Meaning
5. Anxiety as a Condition of Living
6. Awareness of Death and Nonbeing.

WCT is concerned with BSW and how being aware of self and self-worth sets a person up to be true to self and thereby practice affirming their BSW throughout life until they can experience and enjoy RSW. The capacity for awareness of BSW exists and we can be aware of it because it is already affirmed, or we can become aware of the denial of BSW, which infringes on one's ability to feel free to be true to self and also worthy.

We agree that people are free to choose, but that when BSW is denied the person may develop a habit of denying their own self-worth outside of their awareness. Once a person learns that BSW exists and that they have it, they can choose to honor their BSW (be free) and start learning to affirm it. As awareness sets in we can be responsible by affirming self-worth in ourselves and others and perpetuating human dignity for all people.

Striving for identity in WCT includes the uniqueness of each human being. We need courage to discover our core so we can learn how to live from the inside (Tillich, 1952). WCT also suggests that when a client is not true to self but is instead true to the version others place on them, they can experience a lack of personal substance. Existential psychotherapists would have a client consider the possibility that they have become the sum of others' requirements on them. These requirements in WCT become counterfeits, conditions, and injunctions that can cause the client to be what others want them to be to get acceptance or importance in the system but at the price of not having their BSW affirmed while being true to self. Experiencing aloneness is vital for Existentialists because it points to the inability of some individuals to tolerate feeling alone. WCT looks at this as possibly magnified by the feeling of being alone in a system that does not honor BSW and does not make room for someone to be true to self and be worthy.

The idea of relatedness in existential theory is recognized and employed by WCT. The possibility of a neurotically dependent attachment versus a fulfilling interdependent attachment has been adopted by WCT from existential theory. WCT proposes that the later relationship is possible when BSW is affirmed in the system and later by the individual while they are also being true to what is unique about them. The Search for Meaning is important in WCT because it involves personal significance and a sense of purpose. Significance is different from importance in WCT. Importance can be given to a child who accepts conditions and counterfeits to fit in the system. The child who feels important because acceptance is given in the place of affirmed worth is not aware they are trading unconditional significance for importance with conditions. Understanding one's unique significance can be fostered in a system that honors BSW.

Having self-worth gives purpose to an individual living their truth because they can risk discovering their uniqueness and not lose their significance in the family system. In WCT, the psychotherapist will assist the client in identifying how their self-worth needs were not met in their family system, and how unmet self-worth needs can develop into a pattern of denied BSW that becomes pervasive, leaving little room for a sense of overall well-being to be experienced.

References

Akhtar, S. (2016). *Shame: Developmental, cultural, and clinical realms.* London: Routledge https://doi.org/10.4324/9780429480089

Anderson, H. (2003). Postmodern social construction therapies. In T. L. Sexton, G. R. Weeks, & M.S. Robbins (Eds), *Handbook of family therapy. The science and practice of working with families and couples.* New York: Brunner-Routledge.

Badenoch, B. (2023). *The heart of trauma: Healing the embodied brain in the context of relationships.* New York, NY: Norton.

Berger, P. L., & Luckmann, T. (1967). *The Social Construction of Reality: A Treatise in the Sociology of Knowledge.* Garden City, NY: Anchor Books.

Burr, V. (2015). *Social constructionism.* London: Routledge.

Corey, G. (1991). *Theory and practice of counseling and psychotherapy.* Monterey, CA: Thomson Brooks/Cole Publishing Co.

Cozolino, L. (2010). *The neuroscience of psychotherapy: Healing the social brain.* New York, NY: Norton.

Daigneault, D., Brown, C. (2023). Worth-conscious theory: Understanding the role of birthright self-worth and application to clinical practice. *Theory & Psychology, 33*(3), 306–329. https://doi.org/10.1177/09593543221135559

Foster, H. (1983). *The anti-aesthetic: Essays on postmodern culture.* Port Townsend, Wash: Bay Press.

Foucault, M. (1979). *Discipline and punish: The birth of the prison.* Middlesex: Peregrine Books.

Foucault, M. & Colin, G. (1980). *Power/knowledge: Selected interviews and other writings 1972–1977.* New York: Pantheon.

Frankl, V. E. (1992). *Man's search for meaning: An introduction to logotherapy.* Boston: Beacon Press.

Gelso, C. J., & Fretz, B. R. (1992). William James centennial series. *Counseling psychology.* San Diego, CA, US: Harcourt Brace Jovanovich.

Kabat-Zinn, J., Davidson, R.J., Houshmand, Z. (2011). *The mind's own physician: A scientific dialogue with the Dalai Lama on the healing power of meditation.* Oakland, CA: New Harbinger Publications.

Larner, G. (2004). Family therapy and the politics of evidence. *Journal of family therapy, 26*(1), 17–39.

Lewis, M. (1992). *Shame: The exposed self.* New York: Free Press.

Maslow, A. H. (1968). *Toward a psychology of being.* (2nd ed.). New York, NY: D. Van Nostrand Company.

Murdock, N. (2004). *Theories of counseling and psychotherapy: A case approach.* Upper Saddle River, NJ: Pearson Education, Inc.

Porges, S. W. (2011). *The polyvagal theory: Neurophysiological foundations of emotions, attachment, communication, and self-regulation.* New York, NY: Norton.

Rogers, C. R. (1961). *On becoming a person*. Boston: Houghton Mifflin.

Rogers, C. R. (1980). *Way of being*. Boston: Houghton Mifflin.

Sarbin, T. R. (Ed.). (1986). *Narrative psychology: The storied nature of human conduct*. Westport, CT: Praeger Publishers/Greenwood Publishing Group.

Seligman, M. E. (2013). *Flourish: A visionary new understanding of happiness and well-being*. New York, NY: Atria Paperbacks.

Tillich, P. (1952). *The courage to be*. New Haven, CT: Yale University Press.

Vera, H. (2016). Rebuilding a classic: The social construction of reality at 50. *Cultural Sociology, 10*(1), 3–20.

White, M. & Epston, D. (1990) *Narrative means to therapeutic ends*. New York: W. W. Norton.

2
HUMAN DIGNITY AND WELLNESS

Criteria for Wellness

We enjoy a sense of wellness when we can accurately assess our environment through a process called neuroception and determine that our safety is intact (Dana, 2018). As human beings we have an inner system, and we belong to an outer system. Elements in the outer system such as family, work, and community impact how ably our inner system stays well-adjusted. Allostasis, also known as achieving stability through change, is the process by which the body responds to stressors in order to return to homeostasis (i.e., equilibrium; McEwen, 2005). Whereas allostasis represents our body's adaptation process to physical, psychosocial, and environmental stressors, allostatic load is the long-term result of a failed adaptation process resulting in chronic illness or pathology (McEwen & Wingfield, 2003). If the environment changes and additional stressors are felt and persist, a client can experience allostatic overload. This extra load means that more stress hormones are pumped into the body and the body must try to adapt to the new challenge/situation. Allostatic load is akin to a washing machine that continues to run but with the clothes never being cleaned because dirty items are continuously added, and the rinse and spin cycle are stalled. The dirty clothes in the washing machine analogy is similar to the chronic accumulation of stress hormones (i.e., cortisol level) that are experienced in allostatic load. No matter how much our biological wash

 DOI: 10.4324/9781003599739-2

cycle runs, if the stressors are not reduced, the cortisol level remains high and the overloaded and dirty wash cycle will continue. A never-ending and dirty wash cycle in the body can lead to overload and/or burnout.

Wellness consists of eight dimensions that are interdependent: physical, intellectual, emotional, social, spiritual, vocational, financial, and environmental. These dimensions make up a balancing system that requires us to attend to all aspects of wellness or suffer the loss of well-being in one or more dimensions. Wellness, as a multidimensional model, allows us to become our best selves (Ardell, 1999). Self-awareness is considered vital to wellness because with awareness we can pay attention to patterns and learn how we support or disrupt the dimensions of wellness in our own life. We revisit Maslow (1968) to borrow an idea that strikingly adds definition to the worth-conscious theory (WCT) criteria for wellness. Maslow described what we regard as three degrees of valuing others. The first degree includes awareness of the existence of others (e.g., an awareness of strangers without a depth of value for them). The second degree reflects the ability to be cognizant of other human beings as individuals (e.g., to allow the existence of another person to matter). Maslow named this second degree of valuing others as B-cognition, which allows someone to matter to us more than a stranger would. The third degree represents the ability a person has to feel love for another individual, which Maslow named B-love (i.e., being-love). The ability to love another person means we perceive their inherent value and self-worth.

In WCT, the depth of valuing self and others is represented by B-cognition and B-love. We propose that the degrees of valuing self and others are of imminent significance and that doing so honors birthright self-worth (BSW). Maslow's (1968) criteria for wellness is reflected in his list of B-values, which are overlapping facets of being. We appreciate the set of B-values that Maslow (1968) crafted to help us understand what an evolved and mature person looks like when they are fully functioning. Below, we provide the list of B-values and will elaborate on how a few of these B-values inform WCT.

1. Wholeness
2. Perfection
3. Completion

4. Justice
5. Aliveness
6. Richness
7. Simplicity
8. Beauty
9. Goodness
10. Uniqueness
11. Effortlessness
12. Playfulness
13. Truth
14. Self-sufficiency
15. Meaningfulness (added after the 1968 publication of *Toward a Psychology of Being*)

The B-values adopted for the WCT concept of wellness, which encourage the purposeful implementation of WCT include wholeness, justice, goodness, uniqueness, truth, self-sufficiency, and meaningfulness. Following, we provide a definition of each of these seven WCT wellness values. *Wholeness* represents a unity of personal truth and acknowledgement of BSW. Also included in this definition is the ability to embrace the four pillars of self-worth and to experience oneself as contributing to a full life experience as an individual, family, community, and workforce member. *Justice* is defined as adhering to the fair and orderly practice of acknowledging the BSW of all people regardless of difference. Justice also reflects our effort to seek to understand all human beings as worthy. *Goodness* indicates the desirability of healthy functioning, which includes affirming self-worth, building the four pillars of self-worth, and achieving and maintaining RSW. *Uniqueness* is defined as non-comparability such that BSW is bestowed on each human being without diminishing pursuit of "one's" truth as it unfolds overtime. *Truth* signifies our reality that BSW exists, that it can be affirmed or denied, and that denied self-worth is a cause of pathology in human beings. *Self-sufficiency* represents the ability of humans to be environment-transcending. In other words, even if the system they lived in did not consistently affirm their self-worth, persons can learn how to honor their BSW and begin building the four pillars of self-worth independent of their original system. *Meaningfulness* is the recognition of human worth as having a significant purpose in the lived experience of all people. Every individual accepting the endowment of self-worth as a birthright may benefit from a depth of meaning that stems from being worthy.

Worth-Conscious Theory: Wellness Values

To inform the WCT wellness model, we have incorporated seven of Maslow's fifteen B-values. Our selected list of seven wellness values, when present in a system, elucidates how affirming and managing self-worth is essential to well-being. In the WCT wellness model, wellness exists within well-being and well-being cannot endure without affirming self-worth. Maslow (1968) asserted that the B-values are so important to wellness that when they are not adhered to, the experience of suffering and/or pathology is at risk. Moreover, he provided a list of meta pathologies that can arise in the absence of being (B) values. Meta pathologies are less general than standard pathologies and are described by Maslow as a personalized type of mental health malady (i.e., frustration and discontent) that is experienced by individuals who are unable to satisfy their meta needs. According to Maslow (1968), the inability to fulfill meta needs (e.g., specific creative, intellectual, or aesthetic needs) results in meta pathology when B-values are not reinforced. Each of the B-values can be deficient in a client's repertoire of behavior. A client's behavior pattern can have more of these values absent than present, thereby presenting the client with numerous challenges. The following is a condensed list of meta pathologies introduced by Maslow, which are deemed counter to the desired impact of having and fostering values related to well-being: mistrust, disbelief, selfishness, hatred, restlessness, emptiness, hopelessness, surrender, insecurity, anger, disoriented, depressed, strain, over-striving, paranoia, over-dependent, and meaninglessness.

Maslow (1980) believed that we can be value-deprived by our environment which can set us up to suffer from meta pathologies. He further suggested that we can have a sense of unworthiness that frustrates our interest in attaining the highest ideal (e.g., intrinsic values). In WCT, we agree that denied self-worth in the family or larger system can cause hopelessness and lead a person to believe they are unworthy of being known, loved, and respected, and of living their truth. A client's lack of experience with worth-affirming interactions allows meta pathologies to develop. The unintentional switch of having life needs and self-worth needs met and then unmet allows the meta pathologies from denied self-worth to emerge. The absence of a healthy development (i.e., not experiencing self-worth as a birthright nor having it affirmed during formative years) impacts five of the eight dimensions of wellness and all the WCT wellness values. In summary, the five dimensions of wellness that are negatively affected by an external or internalized pattern of denied self-worth are intellectual, emotional, social, spiritual, and environmental. A denied sense of self as worthy effects the identity of the client intellectually, emotionally, socially, and spiritually, if indeed they are spiritual. Environmental wellness is at risk when the client is unable to trust family members or larger systems (e.g., environment) to help them be true to themselves and remain a worthy member. The remaining three dimensions of wellness, which include physical, financial, and vocational, may have a secondary impact on wellness without compromising self-worth. That is, the client can possess a physical difference or disability, experience vocational challenges, and/or financial insecurities and not have their self-worth be disrupted. Although these dimensions of wellness represent broad categories of wellness, the WCT wellness values can help the client construct an individualized approach to well-being.

All seven of the WCT wellness values (i.e., wholeness, justice, goodness, uniqueness, truth, self-sufficiency, and meaningfulness) are negatively affected when BSW is denied by either the client or others in the client's system. When BSW is denied, clients will not feel whole; therefore, wholeness as a wellness value cannot be achieved. Justice is not being provided in the system when self-worth is denied, so the client may recognize that conditions in the system are unjust but not know how to rectify that problem. The system is not creating a model of good/healthy functioning because without affirmed self-worth, the client may be disallowed or unable to build their own pillars of self-worth. The client will lose a vital aspect of uniqueness (to be unique and still worthy) because without BSW they are not being true to self in a system that infringes on or punishes some personal truths. Self-sufficiency is not an easy value to maintain because the client may not have enough awareness of their pattern of denied self-worth to transcend the environment. The final WCT wellness value, meaningfulness, cannot be fully recognized because the challenge of living without BSW can make life meaningless.

The Impact of Impaired Wellness on BSW

Affirming BSW starts at the beginning of life when a child's life needs and self-worth needs are met in their family system. Life needs are met when a client's caregivers provided their basic needs of shelter, food, clothing, and safety. Self-worth needs are specific to WCT but were derived from the idea that humans have higher-level needs which include belonging, self-esteem, and self-actualization. When BSW is affirmed, family members consistently honor individual worth as part of the values that are inherent in that system. When the family system has a set of worth-affirming values, even if they are unwritten, the members will naturally honor BSW and actively seek to respond to both life needs and self-worth needs. WCT recognizes belonging as a need that is fulfilled when BSW is consistently affirmed; this affirmation signifies that the person belongs in the system. In addition to Maslow's higher-level needs (i.e., belonging, self-esteem, self-actualizing), the self-worth needs in WCT are self-awareness, self-respect, self-esteem, and self-confidence, which are inclusive of a self-actualizing experience. In Chapter 4, we define each of these self-worth needs, the pillars they create and the importance of realized self-worth (RSW).

Clients either affirm their self-worth consistently as a well-practiced process of meeting their self-worth needs or they deny it. Denying self-worth needs allows a less desirable process and potentially a pathological pattern to become permanent in that client's repertoire of behavior. The process of denying self-worth needs can become a painful pattern. That pattern can allow for maladaptive behaviors, including meta pathologies to take shape. More specifically, Maslow (1968, 1980) referred to meta needs as the driving needs of self-actualizers (e.g., truth, goodness, uniqueness, wholeness, self-sufficiency to be happy). When self-actualizers are unable to secure or are forced to live without the meta needs that provide a happy life, depression, despair, disgust and alienation manifest, which Maslow referred to as meta pathologies. In WCT, clients are not moving toward self-actualization. As psychotherapists, we help them focus on the solid nature of BSW, the contentedness that congruency between truth and worth allows (a type of happiness), and the ability to develop a worth-conscious mindset. We found usefulness in the B-values (i.e., meta needs) as supporting self-worth as a birthright and the practice of affirming self-worth as a way to build pillars of self-worth over a lifetime, eventually enjoying a personal realization of worthiness through practice. Psychotherapists should be attuned to the pathological pattern that emerges when the being values (i.e., meta needs) that their clients need to live a happy life are nonexistent and when their clients' self-worth needs are consistently denied.

There are several tenets within WCT that explain how BSW is denied. Conditions of worth, counterfeits to realizing worth, injunctions that are intrusive and/or abusive, and intergenerational norms of denying self-worth as a birthright are all tenets of WCT that deny BSW because they prevent understanding self-worth as an inherent and enduring aspect of the human experience. Interpersonal neurobiology (IPNB) provides insight into this phenomenon in that our efforts and strong desire to belong and interpersonally connect can be an impetus to stay connected without an awareness of the benefits or harm that the connection provides (Badenoch, 2023). This lack of conscious awareness allows the requirements in a system that do not serve our worth or truth to shape us.

Whether or not a client is aware of the pattern of denied self-worth needs, the problematic pattern of denying the needs that support BSW can allow for a counterfeit to self-worth to become the focal point of the client's life. This counterfeit is held in place by the meta pathologies unique to that person and their family system. For example, a client raised by a mother who was adept at using a counterfeit to BSW may have been conditioned to support the counterfeit, which was a type of flawlessness. In other words, the client was not allowed to comment on mistakes or flaws in the mother's appearance and/or behavior. This particular counterfeit (i.e., flawlessness) perpetuated the notion that worth was conditional (i.e., in order to be worthy, you could not be flawed). More specifically, the client was not allowed to express their truth about human imperfection. Consequently, the client developed an unrelenting sense of depression (i.e., meta pathology) because they surrendered their truth in a meaningful relationship where a pattern of denied self-worth was precedent. For some clients such as this one, the unrelenting component to depression is a fear that self-worth is not inherent or sustainable. To further clarify, the mother's counterfeit which was imposed on the client is contrary to all seven of the WCT wellness values (i.e., wholeness, justice, goodness, uniqueness, truth, self-sufficiency, and meaningfulness). In addition, when a client is not provided interactions that affirm their self-worth, they can normalize the experience of denied BSW in their family system and then begin to deny it within themselves. Following the self-denial of BSW, the client is prone to taking the worth-denying system with them everywhere they go. Wellness in this situation is absent in the individual because the family system did not recognize their life or self-worth needs, placed conditions on their BSW, and promoted a counterfeit to living worthy that allowed for maladaptive personal pathologies to take shape. Although we have introduced two of the key tenets of WCT (i.e., counterfeits and conditional worth) in this section because of their relationship to BSW, each tenet is described in Chapter 4: Worth-Conscious Theory (WCT) Constructs.

WCT and Client Consciousness

In the WCT model, self-worth, specifically BSW, is the primary concern, but consciousness is a secondary key element in improving client wellness. A client can have BSW and not be aware of or conscious of its importance/existence. It is important to note that awareness is basic recognition that something exists, but consciousness is more complex and requires the individual not only to perceive the existence of a phenomenon, but also to more fully grasp the usefulness of it. Alternatively, a client who was raised in a system that normalized denying the worth of one or more members will experience the denial of BSW, which can be perpetuated outside the family system. This means the client is familiar with worth-denying practices and therefore repetition in new situations may be comfortable. The practice of denying self-worth can become commonplace and eventually internalized without the client becoming conscious of the personal harm. The client can continue to engage in a well-practiced pattern of denying their self-worth long after they leave the system where the double denial originated (i.e., denied self-worth in the system and the establishment of a practice of ignoring the denial of BSW). There are two problems that may develop simultaneously when a client's self-worth needs are denied in childhood. Firstly, the family system that perpetuated the client's denial of BSW (with or without understanding the ramifications of this dynamic) set a precedent that can cause the child to believe their BSW does not exist. Secondly, another requirement can veil the first by not allowing family members to become conscious of their BSW (i.e., acknowledging that the denial of BSW causes emotional pain and suffering). This two-fold phenomenon includes allowing one or more family members to be treated as less than worthy (denied BSW), followed by family members learning to ignore the common practice of denying self-worth in their family system (lack of consciousness of the denied BSW). The message in the family then becomes—do not notice what or who we do not affirm in this system.

When our clients have emerged from a family system where their BSW was denied, and their awareness of their unmet self-worth needs was ignored, disallowed, or even punished by their family system, they may believe they do not have permission to explore their denied BSW. In other words, they should not become conscious of the first unspoken rule, which is the nonexistence of BSW for one or more family members. Even outside the family home and safely within a psychotherapy session, the client may resist becoming conscious (at first) of an enduring family phenomenon that damaged their self-worth. Developing consciousness of an unfair family pattern can still feel off-limits to address due to the client's damaged self-worth. It may take time for the client to release the fear of drawing attention to the destructive pattern that people with positional power around them enabled and even reinforced.

The WCT psychotherapist will introduce the client to the possibility of having BSW that cannot be ignored or disallowed and, therefore, they can consistently affirm their BSW through being worth-conscious. This introduction to being worth-conscious may be disconcerting to the client who has been denied permission to think about an unspoken and seemingly indomitable pattern of denying self-worth. In addition to the client's family system imposing a pattern of ignoring their BSW, the client may have also surrendered belief in their BSW. The client may lack the experience of focusing their awareness on their worthiness or countering the pattern of their BSW being ignored in their smaller and larger systems. This unfamiliar experience may cause the client discomfort as they begin to learn the WCT model. We recognize that in psychotherapy, clients have an opportunity to direct their focus toward their BSW in a purposeful and meaningful way that may be new and even unfamiliar.

It is helpful for the psychotherapist to acknowledge that consciousness is actually a learned process and that different families teach this concept with varying degrees of knowledge and understanding. WCT embodies an expanded definition of consciousness as something more than awareness, which is the initial step. Following, awareness is an ability for introspection, understanding, and application. The next section introduces a theory of consciousness, which proposes that people learn how to be conscious and that a depth of consciousness is a modern-day possibility that we believe is a type of open, active, purposeful, and well-honed perceptive skill. We assert that when clients are able to experience and practice consciousness it is a benefit to their wellness.

The History of Human Consciousness Theory

According to Jaynes (1977), consciousness emerged through the social context of human history as a higher and more complex level of self-awareness. Throughout history, individuals have demonstrated the capacity for introspection but have not always had the opportunity to develop this skill. In considering WCT, we acknowledge the relevance of Jaynes' (1977) *origin of consciousness* theory, which provides a broad psychologically based conceptualization of consciousness and the process by which humans become conscious. Jaynes believed that having consciousness meant having a mind-space where introspection could occur. When the individual experienced applying a new perspective to themselves they could adapt their sense of self and learn about themselves as an individual human being engaging in a process of understanding how to link systemic causes to self (Moore, 2021).

A proponent of Jaynes' model asserted that consciousness can be viewed as a type of super-perception that expands human conception to new levels of adaptability (McVeigh, 2023). Historically, consciousness is regarded as a phenomenon that was transmitted through group members socially rather than through genetics. In the ancient past, socializing included nurturing relationships where stories (language and metaphor) were shared which gave context for the way the mental realm could be understood. McVeigh (2023) introduced the term *metaphoric scaffolding*, which refers to the context of consciousness that has been reinforced over several millennia. Metaphoric scaffolding allows for human beings to enjoy how language and complex mental processing are shaped by the social nature of human beings. The modern-day opportunity to experience a deeper and/or focused consciousness may be due to the development of consciousness, over time, into a sophisticated and useful mental process that encourages individuals to think their own thoughts and to be aware of how those thoughts affect them.

The first human interest or effort to be conscious of self, an individual's volition in decision-making about self, was believed to have happened in early civilization possibly just before the recording of Homer's *Odyssey*, in around 800 B.C. Interestingly, Jaynes (1977) noted that the characters mentioned in the *Odyssey* showed the emergence of being conscious of themselves, something which was less evident in Homer's earlier writings (Moore, 2021). Later, when humans became more comfortably conscious of their inner world, they could wonder about the origin of consciousness and how it manifests in their mind, or anyone else's. Our clients were born during a time in history when consciousness is a more familiar concept for them to entertain. There have been many philosophers, scientists, and theorists who have asked questions about the point of origin of human consciousness partly because there are still unknown facets of the human mind. Like those great thinkers, our clients may want to know more about their capacity for or ability to be fully conscious and how aspects of introspection can be learned.

Psychologist and theorist Julian Jaynes contemplated an answer to the question: *What is the origin of consciousness?* His theory of human consciousness invites us, as human beings who can be aware of ourselves, to continue to learn to develop our own capacity for conscious thought. Jaynes (1986) implored us to teach the next generation about the rich inner experience of having and exploring our own consciousness which he believed informed us daily. To Jaynes, human consciousness is vital to understanding ourselves. Prior to the individual being aware of self as we are today, Jaynes (1993) asserted that ancient people were noble automatons unaware of why they did what they did. Furthermore, people attributed their own thoughts as not belonging to themselves. This experience may have been described as getting direction from the Gods who they believed ruled the lands. This direction from the Gods was received and acted on without critical thought about what it meant, or whether it was good or bad. These ancestors were creatures of habit who followed directions as part of their daily routines (Moore, 2021).

Today, we benefit from the many metaphors (stories) shared over time about human capacity for self-awareness and the depth/focus of conscious thoughts that we hold about ourselves. Our mental-processing skills were noticed and then experienced by earlier generations; some professionals have attempted to map our inner world and more fully understand mentation (mental activity). We have gained knowledge about how our physical and spatial awareness can be used, through language, to represent mentation and map conscious thought. When a person becomes aware of something in their world, they can bring it into their mind and make it conscious. They can look at how they already employ language that represents the reality of how ideas occupy mental space like, "I see that idea more clearly," or "I cannot wrap my head around that concept." Clients can continue to discover how language they already use can help them understand their mental world and the mental activity they engage in. This is a mental-processing shortcut that shows the volition to think about self and gives our thinking depth (Jaynes, 1993).

The following case study illustrates how a client's familiar language can be used to map conscious thought. Matilda was raised in a family system that placed the success of male family members above the value of women. Matilda's father was very successful and had no time to spend listening to his daughter's report of her early school days. She tried thousands of times to grab his attention with her favorite drawings. He thought her interest in art, especially drawing, was silly. He told her to draw something useful and maybe become an architect (i.e., a predominantly male industry). She tried, but could not become the successful man in a man's world that her dad promoted as desirable. Her mother was loving, but adhered to a rigid idea that women are only good to look at and are basically ornamentation for men. She would comfort Matilda by reminding her that, "at least she was pretty," meaning she could be a success if she could get a successful man. Matilda tried to please both her mother and her father, but neither effort increased her awareness of her BSW. In essence, Matilda's BSW was disallowed due to the unspoken rules and rigid requirements in her family system.

Matilda loved her parents, even though they did things that hurt her. She was aware of her love for them and rejected the parts of herself that did not fit their set of rules for being lovable. Without awareness of the unspoken requirements in her family system (i.e., succeed in the way that your father did), she grew up and started adulting using the same set of rules for herself that her parents had used. This made her BSW seem more out of reach. When she found herself at the end of another romantic relationship, she "crashed," a word she used to describe an even greater personal failure that made her feel doomed. Matilda sought psychotherapy because her failed relationship felt overwhelming. She feared that she could not be loved or that certain aspects of her personality were unlovable and unfixable. Over time, she slowly started to learn about having self-worth that can be denied, but not lost. When she talked about her self-worth, early on, she would say, "I think I have it, but I forgot what it feels like." As sessions progressed, she recognized that, as a parent herself, she made sure her small children knew they were worthy. She started to grasp that maybe her parents did not affirm her self-worth because they were unaware themselves. They may have perpetuated a set of rigid rules that actually denied her access to knowing her BSW because that was what had happened to them too.

At one point in psychotherapy, Matilda experienced some self-hatred in session and then challenged the idea that she had BSW because her parents were not unintelligent and would have known that she had worth, if indeed she did have some. It was painful for Matilda to push past the curated lack of awareness about BSW and discover her BSW was not imperceptible to everyone. It was also painful for her to become aware of, and acknowledge, that the people she loved caused her unnecessary pain. Her worth was not gone; it was just systematically denied. She could hate the pattern and not hate her parents. As her awareness of her BSW grew, so did her potential to become conscious of how she was honoring her BSW or not. She learned that she could make purposeful choices by keeping her self-worth in mind. She could then act on those choices, and then assess how well her worth-affirming choices served her mental health and overall wellness. This new process was about one worth-affirming choice at a time, which would help her develop a conscious thought pattern which countered her denial.

The strong mental tether to parenting her own children helped Matilda see her own inner child as worthy too. A worth-conscious language skill set was eventually adopted in her mind-space as more normal and basic. The evidence of this adoption came through the way she talked about her BSW. Matilda was becoming more adaptable and purposeful as she came to understand how her BSW was affirmed (or denied) in the choice of words used with herself and others. She could use language that represented seeing without using her eyes and holding onto something without using her arms because it was happening in her mind. Ideas and situations became clearer in her mind and Matilda was now positioned to see what had blocked her view of her worth. She could now hold her sense of worthiness a little longer in her mental space because consciousness about having BSW was possible. Matilda's mind-space was filling up with language and stories that were worth affirming and she could, with continued awareness, allow herself to open up her heart to her worth.

Focused Consciousness

In WCT, we agree that human beings have volition and can use willpower to engage in thinking about the impact life has on their sense of self. We take this idea further and invite clients to use their volition to focus their ability to be specifically conscious of their BSW. Earlier in the book, we established that self-worth, as a birthright, is a powerful narrative. In addition, we want to further promote the idea that BSW is a component of wellness that, when focused on, can help support one's adeptness in adapting to challenging situations. When a client considers a new way to think or is considering a new thought pattern to adopt, they can become conscious of something new and seek to add it to their repertoire of thoughts, feelings, and actions. Similarly, the addition of new ways of feeling and acting are also true when BSW becomes a focal point of consciousness. The client who begins to consider themselves as worthy, as they should, may find a reservoir of delight at the idea of worthiness that was already a profound experience existing without words. In other words, clients who are seen as worthy by someone in childhood may recognize the experience of feeling worthy in adulthood, but they may not fully understand the experience due to a lack of consistent exposure to a worth-affirming source and therefore they do not have the convenience of words to label it as real and personal.

Some clients may already use language to describe this deep and peaceful reservoir of worthiness that resides within them as something they could see but not always feel, or that they have felt before but did not know how to believe in its constancy. There are more varied statements about how a client's worth occupies their mental space, such as when it is recognized as haveable by a client who may refer to human worth as real but not always easy to understand. Developing a conscious focus on BSW can assist the client in naming the phenomenon and then allowing them to use it as a tool for finding and enjoying self-worth-based wellness.

Clients in modern society may have a degree of consciousness about themselves that does not include BSW because their family narratives evolved without that centering concept. Clients today can become more or differently conscious of themselves with or without focusing their consciousness on affirming their self-worth. However, we maintain that a conscious focus on affirming BSW can make a valuable difference. In other words, clients can further their learning by not just becoming conscious of self but also directing their consciousness toward being worthy. The ability to focus on BSW and allow it to become a tool for health and wellness began with the awakening of consciousness in members of society hundreds of years earlier. It is noteworthy that this conscious focus on BSW allows our clients to center their sense of self and improve their life story. In Jaynes' (1977) research, an individual sense of self further developed once civilizations became established and the ability to think about oneself as existing (i.e., such as what we are doing, how we are doing, and why we do certain things) was more common. We can now add to our shared human story what, how, and why human worth matters to each individual.

As psychotherapists we can utilize a modality, such as family systems theory, that helps clients to differentiate and thereby develop a separate sense of self. What if a type of reintegration is also vital to the whole of human experience wherein an aspect of self as part of a worthy whole does not detract from a person being separate (unique). This can happen in modern society because we can conceive of our mentality as belonging to us and yet recognize it is influenced by others within the systems where we share membership. We can see how we think differently or independently from others and also recognize that some similarities allow us to live together in harmony. Instead of noble automatons with groupthink, we are developing into systemically oriented individuals who are unique and worthy of ourselves and value the advantages of togetherness.

It is important to grasp that worth consciousness, when seen as a universal endowment belonging to everyone, does not take human beings backward to a groupthink experience similar to the pre-conscious era of mindless group participation. A lack of individuation was common in tribal groups because people needed to think and act together in order to survive (Jaynes, 1977). Today, we understand and appreciate the benefit of connectedness and community whilst also remaining on some level independent from others (i.e., self-differentiation; Bowen, 1978). We offer the African proverb "We can go farther together," to further illustrate the importance of connectedness and community. However, in choosing community we must also increase civility for every individual possessing differences that we ourselves may not experience (Afriprov.org, 2000).

Differentiation may not have been an easy option for people before the era of Homer. The emergence of writing as a common practice allowed people to consider themselves as noteworthy of recognition as independent from one another (Jaynes, 1977). This allowed reflexive consciousness to become an option for more and more people to experience. The use of language (reading and writing) allowed people to become more aware of self. As a result of this self-awareness, people could also become aware of the importance they held in their community. The acquisition of new language skills also meant that people could affix labels to one another. Labels came to include the versions we still see clients suffering with today, and which Carl Jung referred to in his work, such as inferiority and superiority.

Clients who are conscious and affirming of their BSW are capable of expanding their consciousness to include self-worth that is both personal and universal. They can apply BSW to any well-being narrative fostered within their family system. They can also counter a dynamic that denies BSW by becoming more worth-conscious. BSW can be a key element in the human story which benefits clients as individuals and as members of the human race. The combination of clients being unique and worthy as individuals and within systems may elevate and equalize their lived experience.

We asked ourselves the following question: why have we not yet made an adjustment to our thinking about human value as being a birthright for all? Is it that something useful in early systems (e.g., being important) took the place of BSW and became the goal of many individuals? Being important is something people can and do strive to achieve. We see evidence of this desire throughout history in literature, such as Romeo in Shakespeare's play. Romeo lacked importance to the family of the woman (Juliet) with whom he was infatuated. He was the wrong sort of person and, no matter what he tried, he could not make himself more important to Juliet's family. The young couple viewed their love as worth the risk of losing family ties because young love can make one forget about the power enforcing the rules. However, the worth of their beloved would never be honored by either partner's family, so they felt doomed to see worth in each other that would never be acknowledged by the larger system. Where there is inferiority or unimportance, BSW is invisible/denied.

WCT proposes that there may have been an original misinterpretation of importance as representing the worth of the individual which was damaging to the individuals who endured a lesser degree of importance throughout history. These people did not have the benefit of being treated equitably and had no recourse in the system. This can occur in smaller family systems as well. Labels of inferiority deny self-worth. The individuals suffering to get out from under such a label may not be allowed to move up because the someone(s) keeping them down may assume that there is little room at the top and so they refuse to make room for more people. Systemically, where there is inferiority there is usually also someone claiming superiority. The favored or more important family member who gets status (instead of worth) may fight to keep their status (superiority) while never feeling worthy. This system error may also set members up to become self-obsessed as they can develop consciousness that is more self-centered in their obsession for positional importance. Their superiority in the system must always be proved and even rewon through competition or domination of others. We also see the development and continuance of a self-centered consciousness that is fixated on positional power in larger systems that perpetuate and preserve systemic inequalities and racism. As such, present-day inequalities in education, employment, wealth, and representation in leadership positions are rooted in a system where one group's claim of superiority is advanced while others are deemed unworthy and inferior.

The misrepresentation of importance as an individual's worth in our WCT model is further explained below. In WCT, a person can engage in important work and enjoy doing something that has importance to them; once the accomplishment is complete, however, the importance stays with the event. The client may feel compelled to repeat acts of importance to feel important themselves, but this is a hamster wheel effect in which the person is pursuing importance because they are not fully conscious of their BSW. The client may be desiring the lift that systemic importance (above others) provides but does not sustain. They can be helped to review the cyclical pattern—that once the pursuer reaches the top of a self-importance wheel, they fall down out of importance again until they achieve something new. Importance, in WCT, is a thing outside of self that is obtained temporarily (it does not add or take away from BSW) but it can become a counterfeit to realizing self-worth because it feels similar to being worthy (significance) without the enduring benefit that affirming self-worth provides. Psychotherapists using WCT to assist a client who is in a pattern of denied self-worth that is complicated by the presence of self-importance as a desired counterfeit, will invite the client to share their history of the cycle of obtaining a sense of superiority and fearing inferiority that has been driving and sometimes directing their decisions. The client and psychotherapist will listen to the story together and start to make a map of where the counterfeit to self-worth shows up, how often it is present, and how powerful that narrative is in the mind of the client and within their family system. We will provide a more thorough explanation in the section on counterfeits later in Chapter 6.

Mindful Cultivation of Consciousness

Mindfulness is a purposeful type of mental exercise that allows a client to rise above self-conscious thinking and into mental space where they can observe all aspects of self without judgment. Blackburn (1999) provided perspective on the separate, but connected mental and physical properties within a human being. He referred to Descartes's philosophy that people are more secure with the knowledge in their own minds and that there is a magic moment when the mind and body collaborate in what we experience—experience which cannot be seen by outsiders. Cultivating the skill to access the mental space where consciousness is free-flowing takes practice. Mindfulness helps clients to get into that space and then observe what is there. One of the goals of mindfulness is to avoid judging any of your thoughts; this includes thoughts about our physical, emotional, experiential, relational, and mental processes. If a client is in the habit of being overly critical or judgmental, they may practice self-conscious thinking and not have awareness of worth-conscious options.

We can be aware of something and yet not fully understand the quality of it. The practice of mindfulness as a consciousness discipline allows us to observe our own mind with empathy and become more conscious of what is there without hating it (Kabat-Zinn, 2003). Labels that have been placed upon us by others limit our access to and acceptance of BSW; therefore, it is crucial that we suspend judgment and not label our thoughts with the good or bad requirements placed on us in childhood but instead assess which thoughts are helpful or unhelpful in our recognition of self as worthy. The practice of mindfulness as a wellness routine can include steps or aspects both from the original Buddhist tradition and also from modern iterations popular in the western world. The Buddhist tradition is concerned with nonmaleficence and equanimity in the mind/heart of the consumer. We recognize the value of cultivating equanimity and disavowing harmful systemic requirements, and furthermore believe that addressing all labels that allow for inferiority or superiority can be part of a mindful practice. In WCT, freeing oneself from the harsh labels of inferiority that allow a client to feel insecure is a psychotherapeutic motive for practicing mindfulness. In essence, we want clients to be free of any systemic labels of inferiority, which can reduce or eliminate self-consciousness as a mental focus. We also hope that with the ability to focus, mindfully, on one's consciousness that the innate nature of self-worth as a birthright can come into focus. Freeing oneself from systemic labels does not make a client feel superior because BSW is not a label that lifts a client above others.

In WCT, self-worth is not just a thought or feeling; it is a quality of being. A quality that is a birthright for all humans. The initial stability of self-worth as a quality takes shape when it is reinforced in the first few years of life by caregivers who invite children to experience having life needs and self-worth needs met. As children grow, they can begin to practice affirming BSW in themselves and in others. With practice, BSW becomes realized (RSW) as belonging within our whole sense of self. WCT acknowledges human worth and being conscious of that worth as a healthy purpose. Mindfulness helps fulfill this purpose by instructing clients to recognize *all* of their thoughts without resistance, which will allow their BSW supporting thoughts to surface.

Scholars have noted that Buddha was able to discover limitless joy through meditation and that he experienced confidence, stability, trust, and clarity of mind once his joy permeated his awareness (Epstein, 2013). In sharing Buddha's experience, Epstein offered us the idea that when we get out of our own way (possibly meaning the labeled self), we discover a more stable self. During a conscious state of mindfulness, a person is both the observed and the observer. A benefit to being both the observed and the observer is the advantage of experiencing ourselves from different points of view, which leads to a more stable, confident, and worthy self. It is believed that a type of joy is recovered in a state of mindfulness (Epstein, 2013).

If mindfulness is a practice that allows clients to become more conscious of their beliefs, they can become conscious of their BSW. A client may enjoy discovering that in the midst of all their positive and negative beliefs, BSW exists unchanged. In WCT, clients who experience their BSW as a quality of being may allow a state of contented joyfulness to emerge. The consciousness of worthiness is more than just an awareness of the existence of self-worth, but rather it is the experience of trusting our BSW that promotes clarity when faced with difficult decisions. When a client values their self-worth, they can build the four pillars of self-worth throughout their life.

An important benefit that a mindful worth-conscious focus can provide to a client is the experience of their sense of self as whole, real, connected, and worthy. During mindfulness, a type of flow can also be achieved, which is an additional benefit where the client can sustain a mental state based in their BSW. In his book *Flow*, Mihaly Csikszentmihalyi (1991) helped us understand that consciousness is not a mysterious process; rather, it results from biological processes. He explained that consciousness emerges from a complicated neurological architecture and that the human conscious mind is self-directed. In other words, a client can choose to override a reflexive response to events, selecting instead a course of action that can include what their senses report but also respond according to a preferred focus. By choosing the contents of consciousness (i.e., selected focus), a person can use their conscious thoughts purposefully to persevere through challenges and overcome obstacles, which Csikszentmihalyi regarded as perhaps the most important trait for enjoying one's life. According to IPNB, clients who do not feel safe or do not know how to trust what is safe in their family system may be triggered into a state of fear or shame and become defensive when talking about how they were denied the things they needed. The profusion of interactions within our primary relationships allows us to gradually internalize and practice what is possible in our neural pathways (i.e., a well-travelled map in the brain), limiting whether we are more dominantly self-conscious or worth-conscious. The dominating pattern of self-conscious or worth-conscious occurs because the limits imposed in our primary system follows us and continues to dominate outside the system. In systems where the truth and worth of its members were valued and supported, worth-consciousness and the members' experience in the system are fostered.

Form and function are represented in the ability that a client has to achieve a conscious state. The form is the brain, and the functional aspect of consciousness involves information about the environment outside and inside the individual. What is happening to the client can be assessed by them and action can be taken (Csikszentmihalyi, 1991). This allows for information about self to be prioritized in a way that we are not only reacting or being reflexive to information, but we can take charge of it. We can make some information matter more, like having a birthright.

WCT included the idea of consciousness and specifically applied it to the possibility of sustaining a worth-conscious focus within the client's state of mind. The intention of helping clients become worth-conscious is to support their wellness and promote a universal potentiality that the human story can include the BSW of all people. Everyday events, including our thoughts, feelings, and actions, can be highlighted intentionally with a conscious focus to support self-worth. A state of worthiness can be experienced consistently through flow and maintained with practice.

References

Afriprov.org (2000). Luo proverb, Weekly African Proverb, Dec. 21st. Rev. Joseph Healy Moderator. https://afriprov.tangaza.ac.ke/2000-weekly-african-proverbs/

Ardell, D. B. (1999). Definition of wellness. *Ardell Wellness Report, 18*(1), 1–5.

Badenoch, B. (2023). *The heart of trauma: Healing the embodied brain in the context of relationships.* New York, NY: Norton.

Blackburn S. (1999). *Think: A compelling introduction to philosophy.* New York: Oxford University Press.

Bowen, M. (1978). *Family therapy in clinical practice.* New York: Aronson.

Csikszentmihalyi, M. (1991). *Flow: The psychology of optimal experience.* New York, NY: Harper Perennial.

Dana, D. (2018). *The polyvagal theory in therapy: engaging the rhythm of regulation.* (1st ed.). New York: W.W. Norton & Company.

Epstein, M. (2013). *The trauma of everyday life.* New York, NY: The Penguin Press.

Jaynes, J. (1977). *The origin of consciousness in the breakdown of the bicameral mind.* Boston, MA: Houghton Mifflin.

Jaynes, J. (1986). Consciousness and voices of the mind. *Canadian Psychology/Psychologie Canadienne, 27*(2), 128–148. https://doi.org/10.1037/h0080053

Jaynes, J. (1993). *The origin of consciousness in the breakdown of the bicameral mind.* London: Penguin Books. (original work published in 1977).

Kabat-Zinn, J. (2003). Mindfulness-based interventions in context: Past, present, and future. *Clinical Psychology: Science and Practice,* 10(2), 144–156. https://doi.org/10.1093/clipsy.bpg016

Maslow, A. H. (1968). *Toward a psychology of being.* (2nd ed.). NY: D. Van Nostrand Company.

Maslow, A. H. (1980). *The farther reaches of human nature.* New York, NY: Penguin Books.

McEwen, B. S. (2005). Stressed or stressed out: What is the difference? *Journal of Psychiatry and Neuroscience, 30*(5), 315–318.

McEwen, B. S., & Wingfield, J. C. (2003). The concept of allostasis in biology and biomedicine. *Hormones and Behavior, 43*(1), 2–15.

McVeigh, B. J. (2023). Consciousness as "Super-perception." *Julian Jaynes Society Spring Newsletter,* https://www.julianjaynes.org/2023/07/12/consciousness-as-super-perception/

Moore, J. W. (2021). They were noble automatons who knew not what they did: Volition in Jaynes' the origin of consciousness in the bicameral mind. *Frontiers in Psychology, 12,* 811295. https://doi.org/10.3389/fpsyg.2021.811295

3

CONGRUENT SENSE OF SELF

Self-Worth and True Self

The ability to communicate one's personal experience openly and honestly to other people is vital to feeling worthy. Authentic self-disclosure (i.e., truthfulness about oneself) is regarded as conducive to a healthy personality (Jourard & Landsman, 1980). In worth-conscious theory (WCT), we propose that a client's truth, no matter how well received in shared systems, needs to be lived and shared as part of the worth-affirming process. One's lived and shared personal truth that can be safely experienced is crucial to honoring birthright self-worth (BSW). The experience of self-worth as a birthright means that a human being has worth that can be affirmed individually and systemically. Having truth about oneself that is openly and honestly known by the individual and safely shared with others, without losing loving-kindness, affirms that the person is worthy to be their authentic self. For example, a client whose depression reportedly started in childhood, recalled being athletic and enjoyed participating in sports and music programs; however, he was told by his parents to choose one over the other. When pressure was put on him to choose sports, especially football, he followed the requirement imposed by his family system. He remembered that his parents loved his obedience, but as he reflected on this event as an adult client, he felt less worthy. The truth he had shared about his love of music fell on deaf ears. During his

 DOI: 10.4324/9781003599739-3

middle school years, when he cried after a rough practice because he had been hit harder than usual, he told his parents he wanted to quit. At first, he was told that quitting was for losers and there was no place for losers in their family. He reluctantly agreed to stay in the sport another year and his sadness deepened. He did not tell anyone that he would hang outside the orchestra room listening to the music he longed to create himself. He kept it a secret because it had become a truth his family could not love. The question we ask in WCT is when does a person/client know what their truth is, and when does knowing their truth and not living it start to make self-worth conditional.

When a client has truth about themselves that they are reluctant to share with others because it will not be welcomed or appreciated, the client is unintentionally pushed to move against their own self-worth. This problem is difficult to remedy in psychotherapy if the client's denial or reluctance to share their truth is due to self-protection from a system that is hostile toward a truth that they experience. The client may resist being open about a known truth even in a safer environment, like in session, because they may have developed a habit of denying an unacceptable truth, even though it is a truth that cannot be uninhabited. On top of the habit of defending a secret and denying their truth, they may have heard dismissive or aggressive statements made by family members that demean people experiencing a similar truth. This dynamic of family members expressing verbal or emotional aggression about a difference that is unacceptable in the family system sends a powerful message to any member that might not be fully conforming. An additional impact this rigid system requirement may have on a member who has a lived truth that is labeled as unacceptable in their family is that they may hide the truth or rebel against the system to not lose their self-worth.

Not living a known truth to make other family members comfortable can cause a client to feel unworthy both within themselves and within the system where their truth is unwelcome. The longer the client must endure conforming to systemic requirements that deny their truth the more worth-denying thinking may occur. Once a habit of worth-denying thinking takes shape the client's mental health may become negatively affected. The client may look at the world and the diversity that exists and ask: Why is my difference an intolerable difference to the people who I thought loved me? The client may suffer from a complicated combination of having self-worth affirmed only when conforming and thereby develop a habit of denying their truth to fit in. Family members are made more comfortable by the client who slowly loses their lived truth in exchange for conditional love. In doing so, the client experiences conditional worth and the family's love for the client becomes a weapon of conformity.

Conforming in order to be loved is not one of the seven WCT wellness values. In fact, it can interfere with all seven values and therefore deserves a special mention as a behavior that can become pathological because the true self can be lost. There are probably thousands of ways a person can conform to fit in; however, the desire to fit in is not problematic on its own. Conforming may become pathological when the person trying to fit in has to give up aspects of themselves that are vital to their whole sense of self. Wanting to belong is a common and healthy human desire. The neuroscientist John Cacioppo stated that because loneliness can be a disabling condition, it compels us to pursue relationships with others as a fundamental element for well-being (Seligman, 2013). Conformity itself is not necessarily problematic as any large organization, such as a prison system, will require conformity to rules and regulations that promote order, reduce problems, and uphold the safety of its workers and members. A misapplication of systemic conformity to increase a type of safety in the system could be instigated in a family system when, for example, one parent experiences a lack of emotional safety because their child does not conform to the expected personal standard that the parent holds. This can result in two or more family members experiencing competing values. Seligman (2013) stated that values are different from ethics. Whereas ethics refers to standards of right and wrong that govern a person's behavior, values reflect our beliefs and what we care about. In other words, what we value influences how we behave. We agree and will add that values are also different from personality characteristics and that when we care about something to the point that we value it—it can become dominant in our decision-making process. Although we are less clear as to why someone might experience their values as an extension of themselves (i.e., personality trait), we do understand that when a person has accepted a set of values as their own, they feel wounded when what they value is disregarded by others. In WCT, we recognize that humans have values and that a set of values may be as unique as the individuals who hold them. The concern we have is not that different sets of values exist, but that someone can value compliance to their values so strongly that they deny the self-worth of others. This can happen to lesser or greater degrees. The following story is one of lesser weight in the overall outcome, but still one where values compete, and one person's self-worth is on the line.

Competing values and parental authority over what is valued in the system can take precedence over respecting differences. In a particular family system one child (who for the sake of this example is female) may be required to carry on as the next owner of the family business. First, the child does not want to be required to take over the family business. Second, the family business is a sandwich shop and, due to dietary requirements, the non-conforming child is a vegan. So, if she must take over the shop, she wants to make some changes. The child, now a young adult, may be seen as rebellious because she has competing values about what has traditionally been how the family business is run. The argument, however, was primarily focused on what could or could not be included on the sandwich menu at the shop. When the young adult was given an increase of love by her parent for making a conforming choice, which was to put off making a decision, love then becomes the parent's tool to get a preferred outcome. In this example, the parent needs sameness/conformity to feel safe. Moreover, the young adult child noticed, over time, that in some instances parental love was not a message about her truth but rather a direct contradiction of her truth. In other words, she is good enough to run the family business but not worthy of her reality, which includes adding items to the menu that do not cause food allergies in support of her vegan status.

Below we apply the WCT wellness values to address the existence of two worthy people having competing values. In WCT, we acknowledge that both individuals have personal truth and BSW (i.e., wholeness). Their differences are reflected in the value and cost they place on the menu items, but they both remain equally worthy and can still love each other. Their differences do not make one person wrong, and an effort to incorporate items they both value could be helpful (i.e., justice). When competing values exist, they are not compared to decide which set is better, or whose values win. Instead, the individuals can look at the pros and cons of each value and determine why it is meaningful and useful to the person who holds it dear (i.e., goodness & meaningfulness). The desire to understand the other person's inclusion of a value that is not as important within one's own set of values allows for individuality (i.e., uniqueness). The truth of both people is heard, and their different set of values does not detract from their BSW (i.e., truth). If each individual can allow for the different sets of values to co-exist by leaning into what is worth affirming, they may be able to bridge the gap of misunderstanding between them and transcend the competition mindset to make room for what can work (i.e., self-sufficiency). Transcending the 'stuckness' of competing values can be achieved when the acceptance of each other as worthy and different is desired, and through clarifying what is being accepted and by whom. It is important to understand that WCT does not expect one to accept another's truth as something they understand or experience themselves. Accepting another person's truth that is not personally understood means that we are *trusting the person* who is experiencing congruency due to feeling worthy while living their truth. In the example above, the parent cannot easily accept something about their daughter that is not within them. WCT would not encourage the parent to torture themself by considering what it would be like to be in her shoes because what would be a choice for the parent is a reality for the daughter. Understandably, the parent may be unable to lean into personal experiences and fully appreciate the difference they question, but the parent can *trust their daughter's* understanding of herself and embrace the congruency that is created by her combined honesty and worth. More simply stated, it is the daughter's truth that she is vegan, and her parent can accept that the daughter has an understanding of herself that is real such that when she is experiencing congruency in that reality (i.e., honesty/authenticity) and worthiness, she is better situated for healthiness and wholeness.

We invite our readers to apply the WCT wellness values when exploring the many facets of a client's identity, especially the elements that are an integral part of their wiring that make them feel different in their family system. Clients with a lived truth (e.g., lesbian/gay, asexual, bisexual, transgender, queer, etc.) that impacts their acceptance in the system and may erode their will to live, may suffer the inequity of competing values in their family or community that deny their worth by dominating what can be valued. Those clients can have their BSW reinforced and engage in worth-affirming conversations in psychotherapy about how their truth is part of their overall wholeness and therefore increases their wellness. The goal will be to eventually have healing conversations outside of psychotherapy sessions with family members who are willing to gain perspective on how to honor the self-worth of others who have a different set of values that are equally personal to them. The competition between who is right can turn into a collaboration about the worthiness that is bestowed to everyone.

Psychotherapists can also consider the advantage of accepting people who have differing preferences that are not intrinsic to identity. Certainly, people we care about may have other competing values that do not influence their will to live. Neither party needs to lose their sense of worthiness because of competing values (e.g., pro-choice or pro-life, Democratic or Republican, religious or non-religious, etc.) that exist amongst their family members. WCT encourages applying the same worth-affirming process of believing the family member who is seeking congruency through identifying with a cause they value. The process would focus on affirming one's self-worth even when you don't understand or value their cause.

True Self and Trust

Competing values can add to the challenges in relationships with others, and they can also interfere with the relationship we have with ourselves. You can still trust a family member who has a different set of values from yours when the family member is consistent about what they value, even if you do not like their different set of values. On the other hand, if what you have been told to value (value hand-me-downs) and what you determine to value are in conflict, you may experience an internal divide, which potentially interferes with the ability to trust yourself. Being true to the set of values we were given may disallow a client from being true to the set of values that make them feel worthy. The ability to recognize what a lack of trust feels like in the mind and body is helpful in being true to ourselves. To belong to a system, especially one we are born into, is to be included before we are fully known by the other members. Weininger (2022) invited us to consider that being able to trust ourselves and others enhances our ability to experience interconnectedness and that belonging is vital in healthy human experience. Trust as an experience of belonging is developed over time and includes emotional identification with those who have shared values and experiences (Anderson et al., 2021).

One of the oddities about trust is that it is almost always given a positive connotation, but occasionally we encounter someone who trusts that the person who did them wrong will do so again, if allowed. So, in that case, trust is about consistency. Could it be that once we are capable of recognizing the pattern of behavior that a certain set of values evokes in the person who holds the values, we then evaluate how consistently that person lives by their set of values in order to trust them? Perhaps as we are getting to know someone, we try to discern what they value so as to better know what to trust about them. Like trusting a vampire will hunt at night or that a violinist will need to practice daily to achieve what they value. It is possible that a combination of nature and nurture is present for the inclusion of certain values. In other words, we may be presented with values that begin within us and are about our nature (i.e., inherent characteristics we are born with), and some values may come from outside of us and reflect how we were nurtured (e.g., acquired characteristics we adopt). To further clarify, examples of inherent characteristics include valuing gender, sexuality, physicality, temperament, and aspects of personality such as those represented in the Big Five personality traits: openness, conscientiousness, extroversion, agreeableness and neuroticism. Examples of acquired characteristics that we adopt include valuing being faithful or faithless, forgiving or unforgiving, hopeful or hopeless, kindness or unkindness, cooperativeness or competitiveness to name a few. Valuing BSW can be a result both of nature and of nurture. Whereas inherent or acquired values can reinforce BSW, acquired values could deny or replace the significance of BSW and create a counterfeit to having self-worth as a birthright, such as when gaining power (i.e., acquired value) in a system is more important to an individual than the balance that benefits and acknowledges the BSW of all members in the system.

For someone who is interested in personal growth, we suspect that there is likely some level of difficulty involved in incorporating a new value into an already established set of values. More precisely, psychotherapy clients have demonstrated how incredibly challenging it can be to add a value, especially one that is not handed down from family, into their personal set without engaging in introspection and deliberation about why they feel compelled to make a major addition to their set of values. The decision to add a new or different value than what the family system has already declared as important to their established set of values can be a painstaking process about what will help the client in determining how much they trust what they value. During deliberation they may begin to see a gap in their set of values that excluded self-worth as a birthright. The client could recognize that they believe in self-worth, but that it was a distant idea in their family system rather than a priority of conscious thought. If the client was not encouraged to live from their BSW and see it as a priority in their decision-making, it may be alien to see the advantages of honoring BSW as an adult.

In consideration of the nurture variable as related to how we learn to value and trust, we offer the following explanation. If we belong in a system before we are fully known, and our true nature develops into a difference that is rejected by one or more members in the system, then conformity to the systemic requirements could mean survival. Consequently, survival becomes a value that competes with one's true identity. The child accepting this counterfeit for having BSW may feel the competition playing out in their minds and hearts as they want to survive and yet also want to be who they are. When the unconditional acceptance of worth we are bestowed in the first few years of life is altered to conditional acceptability, we may not understand why things changed but feel compelled to accept that we must change to remain acceptable. We may remember feeling the benefit of unconditional acceptance in our early years and then feel confusion about why conditions of worth that uphold a counterfeit were introduced. The confusion could spur a deeper message in childhood about the shift away from unconditional worth—*am I not worthy* (without conditions) could be a question that turns into a self-fulfilling prophecy later in life. Kantor (2000) shared that an argument that has high stakes can take place between people where one person is unwilling to give an inch because it feels like they are standing their ground (honoring their values) by saying, "Here's who I am; my identity, my very being is at stake."

In WCT, we encourage our clients to look at both values of nature and nurture in order to prioritize which values support their inherent self-worth and align with their lived truth. This means that clients can discover their true nature and therefore become able to value what is inherently unique about them, but that only happens after they have already learned a set of acquired values that may or may not affirm their BSW. In other words, if any of the inherent values in a person seemingly move against the set of values already established in the family, it can feel like a type of mutiny. The child who needs to value something that is unique to them but uncommon in the family system may feel like a disruptor. If they are not allowed to simultaneously live their present truth and remain accepted in the system, the competition about which values are allowed may tear apart the family or the child, depending on which values win (nature versus nurture). The antidote is a combination of nature and nurture values, which allows differences that develop for one member to be considered and included because the BSW of each member is recognized. When the families' set of acquired values was taught by trusted nurturers and the lesson included adherence to the acquired set of values by the children in the family, clients may trust the requirements in the system over their own sense of self. Knowing when values of nature have a significant advantage over nurture-based values can assist clients in aligning with their personal truth. Clients do not have to discard the acquired values but can take an inventory of the systemically approved values and determine which ones align with their inherent nature (worth & truth). In doing so, clients are better equipped to manage: (a) family members' challenge of and dislike for their inherent values; and (b) the family system's required adherence to an acquired set of values that compete with their lived truth. Prioritizing inherent values and recognizing acquired values that honor BSW help us trust ourselves. Engaging a worth-affirming set of values consistently in our daily decision-making is one of the main goals of WCT. Once the set of values we choose affirms BSW consistently, decision-making about honoring self-worth is lucid.

Competing Values and Trust

In the last section, we introduced the phenomenon of family members having values that can be in competition for relevance in the system. We will expand on that concept by explaining the vulnerability that exists for one or more members in the system when they risk blindly trusting the system's established set of values. More precisely, although a set of values followed consistently can make trusting easier, the trust placed in the established set of values to serve everyone can make one person more vulnerable in the system than other members. The vulnerability of a member may increase when the set of values being used does not serve their lived reality. Anderson et al. (2021) reported that the ability to trust involves a human element and a conviction that others will do what is right, thereby allowing for cooperation between two parties to supersede the uncertainty that trust is beneficial in the system. When a family member presents differently from their family system's preferred and acquired set of values, there is an uncertainty that they experience, which can be explained by a lessening of acceptance and their BSW no longer being honored. The system's preferred values may include some values inherent to the parents that do not fit the lived reality of one or more of the children. The fear of not belonging unless the difference the child is experiencing is hidden, causes the child to feel more vulnerable to rejection. The fear of not feeling valued by others creates a state of vulnerability such that someone living their truth may have to risk being rejected by those they love in order to stay aligned with their personal truth.

A client, who we will call Freddie, may have enjoyed years of full acceptance in the family system until he started to show feminine preferences. He was simply liking the things he liked, which included going shopping with his sisters and modeling the new clothing they would bring home. When his mannerisms started to mimic those of his sisters, his dad pulled him aside and told him he was spending too much time with the girls. He loved hanging out with his sisters and liked that he could be himself with them, but he felt his dad becoming increasingly frustrated with him. He did not think he was doing anything wrong, and yet his dad seemed to reprimand only him when he and his sisters and their girlfriends were all giggling or being silly.

Freddie, being true to his nature and valuing characteristics that make spending time with his sisters easy and enjoyable, was launched into a clash of competing values between himself and his dad. What his dad did not understand is that what would be a choice for him (to accept that his son has an inherent value he is unfamiliar with) was not a choice for his son (experiencing his truth and accepting it). His father had different inherent values such as, men must always behave manlike, or maleness has limited expression. Different acquired values were also expressed by his father, including do not embarrass your parents, and femininity is weak. This set of values was a combination of lived and chosen values which can get tangled up to the point that the person may not remember

which values were chosen by them and which for them. The fact that
Freddie's newly experienced inherent value was never experienced by his
father made Freddie's values seem alien. His father misinterpreted the
inherent value as something that could be stopped instead of recognizing that a request or demand to stop it was an act of rejection of his son.
Unfortunately, his father insisted that Freddie follow the set of values that
prevented a male family member from behaving in ways that could be
labeled as feminine. Freddie had to decide if he could surrender his newly
experienced sense of self, and instead trust his father's set of values over
his own so as to reduce the risk of losing acceptance in the family system.
However, trusting his father's wisdom put him at risk of not adhering
to his own inherent values (maleness does not have limited expression)
that naturally developed as part of his true sense of self. In this situation, trusting his father is not the same as trusting that his father's set of
values will serve his wellness. Freddie is more vulnerable by just trusting his father, wholesale, because if his father's love and support include
conditions placed on Freddie such that he is only worthy when complying, then when he accepts his father's set of values outright, Freddie is in
danger of losing his integrity. When Freddie could not make a distinction
about who or what was being trusted, and how competing values created vulnerability about not belonging where he had always belonged, he
hated himself for being a problem. Hating himself was easier than hating his father because Freddie valued and accepted the differences in his
father. Once Freddie surrendered being himself around his father, he was
left with the reality that competing values in his family demanded a loser.

In exploring the nature side of which inherent values are included,
WCT proposes that to survive as a human being we are wired to signal
others for support before we know what we are doing. As infants, we feel a
sensation in our bodies and send a signal to our caretakers that something
is happening. When a caretaker responds to our hunger signal by feeding
us, we learn to trust our ability to signal what we are really experiencing.
Similarly, when our caregivers respond by fulfilling the need consistently,
we learn to trust their support. Feeling and signaling what is real in our
bodies is hard-wired. When what we need is felt, communicated, and
then reciprocated, we learn that listening to what is real for us is important to our survival. In turn, we learn in the first few years of life that

being vulnerable is respected in the system. We start out being vulnerable and learn to trust that our needs matter to other people in the system where we belong. The support that is available to us as an individual is abundant in the early years and can remain abundant in the resources that we come to value, such as awareness, respect, esteem, and confidence building, as we better discern who we are as an individual. The ability to trust begins as our earliest needs are met (nature) and can expand when we are taught acquired values (nurture), which give us structure until we can be consciously true to our natural inherent values. From there, we may need to assess the whole set of values and choose to keep some of the acquired values that support our personal truth. As psychotherapists, we can support the notion that as humans we can value having our life needs and self-worth needs met. We can guide a client to appreciate that a set of values, which includes the acquired values of others was most likely taught by caretakers to give us guardrails and signposts through life. We can promote an appreciation for caretakers who wanted to teach us from a set of values which made sense to them and also inspire client discernment about how to implement those lessons in a way that does not take away from learning for themselves what inherent values make them unique. As we honor client self-worth, we help them assess which values to keep, and which values they need (inherent) or want (acquired) to remain worthy and true to their sense of self. Clients' assessment of their values includes awareness of what they already have, respect for which values work and why, esteem for values that help them like themselves and the world, and confidence in their choices, or in the ability to learn from making worth-affirming choices.

References

Anderson, E.L., Considine, L., & Patterson, A.S. (2021). The power–trust cycle in global health: Trust as belonging in relations of dependency. *Review of International Studies*, 47(4), 422–442. https://doi.org/10.1017/S0260210521000346

Jourard, S. M. & Landsman, T. (1980). *Healthy Personality: An approach from the viewpoint of humanistic psychology*. (4th ed.). New York: Macmillan Publishing.

Kantor, D. (2000). *My lover, myself: Self-discovery through relationship*. New York, NY: Riverhead Books.

Seligman, M. E. P. (2013). *Flourish*. New York: Simon & Schuster.

Weininger, R. (2022). *Deep Trust: Finding our footing in a turbulent world*. Tricycle Magazine. https://tricycle.org/article/trust-in-ourselves/

4
WORTH-CONSCIOUS THEORY (WCT) CONSTRUCTS

Definition of WCT Terms

Foundational Concepts

Birthright Self-Worth (BSW): The inherent value that exists within all human beings that can be honored by others. All children have BSW and can experience it, with support, until they can become self-affirming and co-create a worth-affirming pattern.

Worth-Conscious: Believing oneself to be worthy as a human being and demonstrating capacity to understand the equity of human worth in varied interactions in order to support one's BSW both individually and interactionally.

Self-Conscious: Believing oneself to be less than worthy in situations, which causes feelings of discomfort.

Life Needs: The most basic needs for physical existence that are based on Maslow's hierarchy of needs: food, water, clothing, shelter, sleep, and physical safety.

Self-Worth Needs: The most basic experiences of humans that allow for learning about individual worthiness by signaling their needs and having their needs attended to in a system with BSW-affirming members.

DOI: 10.4324/9781003599739-4

Realized Self-Worth (RSW): Self-worth that arises from the practice of affirming BSW in cooperation with one's lived truth and therefore becomes stable because it can withstand doubts, fears, failures, and fallibility.

Lost-Worth Story: The story we tell ourselves which keeps us in a pattern of denying our BSW.

Self-Worth Story: The worth-affirming life-script written for us by members of our family system and/or rewritten by us about who we are, how we have differentiated, lived our truth, and remain worthy.

Inherent Values: Valuing inherent characteristics that make you feel like you.

Acquired Values: Valuing ideology or beliefs passed down in the family system.

Competing Values: When a personal (inherent) value competes for importance against a systemic (acquired or inherent for others) value(s). The personal/inherent value that is significant to the individual, may be opposed by the system because it is unfamiliar or unsupported in the system.

Internal Competing Values: Two or more different values held by an individual as equally important which are in opposition and cause internal strife as the individual struggles with the decision of which value is necessary even if it means loss of self or system.

Systemic Exigencies: Demands, conditions, injunctions, and the pursuit of a counterfeit as a requirement of acceptance in the family or larger system.

Intrusive Injunctions: Directions from parents that create conditions that prevent a child from experiencing acceptance, which coincidentally denies BSW. The child will learn to accept conditional worth and not know how to affirm their BSW. Instead of being allowed to be true to themself, the child is taught how to affirm the conditions required in the family system (e.g., the family's version of success).

Abusive Injunctions: Abusive statements in the form of directions or judgments that require a child to conform to conditions that deny their BSW, setting up a pattern of self-denying their worth. The developing truth of the individual may be the target of the abuse.

Worth-Conscious Theory (WCT) Wellness Values: wholeness, justice, goodness, uniqueness, truth, self-sufficiency, and meaningfulness. These seven core values are the substructure for the development of concepts within WCT.

Pillars

Four Pillars of Self-Worth: The worth-affirming pillars we build on a BSW base, which eventually support the development and maintenance of RSW.

Self-Awareness Pillar: The ability to focus attention toward, and attach value to, a forming identity. This includes the ability to examine and clarify our own behavior and develop insight.

Self-Respect Pillar: The ability to focus on protecting the value we experience when BSW is affirmed. This includes setting and maintaining boundaries that support us becoming ourselves.

Self-Esteem Pillar: The ability to focus on the individual value we experience in a BSW-affirming system. This includes recognizing qualities we esteem in ourselves that affirm our BSW.

Self-Confidence Pillar: The ability to trust in the valuation of self as honest. This includes knowing that we have BSW and are worthy of being true to ourselves as we also are becoming a realized self.

Imitation Pillars: Built with conditions that serve a counterfeit, which oftentimes promotes the specific condition of working for worth in a system.

Counterfeits: Any goal in the system that requires the repeated use of conditional building blocks to make imitation pillars. Subsequently, the imitation pillars uphold the goal as more important than BSW. Acceptance in the system is conditional on achieving the goal instead of encouraging the development of realized self-worth.

Worth-Affirming: Moments when BSW is avowed.

Building Blocks: Specific thoughts/words/actions that provide a resource to build one of the four pillars of self-worth or an imitation pillar.

Worth-Denying: Moments when BSW is made to seem unreal or unimportant.

Conditional Worth: Conditions in a system that allow a person to have worked for worth, or worth that is in service of a counterfeit goal (e.g., achievement), or worth that partially affirms BSW with exceptions.

Conditional Building Blocks: Blocks that keep conditional worth in play.

Developmental Stages in Worth-Conscious Theory: Five stages that range from birth through adulthood which align with Erikson's Psychosocial Stages. The Four Pillars of Self-Worth are co-constructed between caregivers and children. BSW can be affirmed through each stage as the child develops their true sense of self by experiencing the pillars below.

Stage One: self-awareness pillar

Stage Two: self-respect pillar

Stage Three: self-esteem pilar

Stage Four: self-confidence pillar

Stage Five: during adolescence, the child begins to accept or reject the building blocks they have been given by caregivers as they work to confirm their identity.

Quadrants

Four Quadrants: The four different possible outcomes of the intersection of life needs and self-worth needs being supported (or not) in a family or larger system. The quadrants are arranged from low to high level of support for both life and self-worth needs.

Quadrant 1 (Q1): The experience of not having self-worth needs affirmed with the additional challenge of life needs not being met at a sustaining level.

Quadrant 2 (Q2): The experiences of not having enough resources to meet life needs consistently but having self-worth needs met.

Quadrant 3 (Q3): The experience of having life needs met or exceeded, but not having self-worth needs met due to the use of intrusive or abusive injunctions that support the conditions of worth in the system.

Quadrant 4 (Q4): The experience of having self-worth needs met effortlessly, while having life needs easily met or exceeded.

Migrating to Q4: The ability to recognize and alter our course with the goal of moving toward a life within Q4 because we understand the importance of having worth-affirming relationships with self and others. Living in Q4 provides opportunity to rewrite our self-worth story to meet our life needs and our self-worth needs at a more beneficial level.

WCT Constructs with Examples

Birthright Self-Worth (BSW)

A birthright can be defined as a privilege possessed at birth. It can be either a natural or a moral right (Serrani, 2022), but it wasn't always recognized as something fairly gifted to everyone. Although the term still exists in some of the oldest religious traditions, it is not necessarily a common practice in modern times. Traditionally, birthright was based on the birth order of one's children. The bestowal of birthright allowed the oldest male child to receive more, often double the property, than the other children (Deuteronomy 21:17 Hebrew Bible/Torah). WCT is not concerned with the bestowing of property or the religious origin of the term birthright; rather, we apply the concept of birthright to extend the privilege of possessing self-worth to all people regardless of status in the system.

Self-worth as a birthright is commonplace in some family systems. We believe that affirming BSW increases systemic and individual wellness while also thwarting a type of psychological pain, "psychache" (i.e., mental/emotional pain from an unbearable condition or reality; Shneidman, 1993, p. 51). Families who understand the positive impact of having self-worth affirmed for each individual member will perpetuate the idea of worthiness even in the face of adversities. Families experiencing the harsh realities of life in Q2 affirm the worth of members even when they cannot afford financially to meet their needs. For example, consider the young adult male who experienced his family going through hard times in which he occasionally was only served popcorn for dinner. He never felt unworthy of a good meal and his parents did not shame him for existing and having needs they could not consistently fulfill. The family practice of acknowledging the BSW of every member, even when the larger community was uninterested in in their plight, reinforced the existence of something inherent that life's challenges cannot reduce or remove from a person. The struggle to have value in the larger system does not prove that a family deserves the hardship they struggle with. Notably, BSW is inherent in all persons and central to working with our clients using a WCT lens. The seven WCT wellness values that are embodied in BSW (i.e., wholeness, justice, goodness, uniqueness, truth, self-sufficiency, meaningfulness) are detailed below.

> *Wholeness*: A sense of wholeness includes one's inner connection with self as worthy and one's relational connection in a system as a valued member. If a client's self-worth is not affirmed, the client will struggle with feeling a sense of wholeness. This lack of wholeness will negatively impact their well-being and possibly alter their overall life satisfaction. Self-worth provides a buffer against distress and emotional upset, thereby promoting one's well-being and life satisfaction (Crocker et al., 2006; Svedberg et al., 2016). When a client's BSW is affirmed by their family of origin, community, or another connection such as the counseling process, a sense of wholeness can be restored.

> *Justice*: Having self-worth denied feels confusing and unjust to a client. Sevig et al. (2000) stated that self-worth is innate without regard to race, gender, age, religion, or physical ability. When a client experiences this injustice, they may erroneously believe their self-worth is lost. Seeing self-worth denied in others may also create confusion and a sense of injustice. The remedial process involves a fair appraisal of the client as having BSW, *just because*.

> *Goodness*: Having self-worth affirmed feels good mentally, emotionally, psychologically, and spiritually. Fukuyama and Sevig (1999) stated that a connection to a higher power can provide a foundation for self-worth. Friedrichs (2016) stated that self-worth is grounded in dignity and does not have to be earned. A client can tap into a healthier (or healing) mindset by engaging in a BSW affirming practice that includes the four pillars of self-worth.

> *Uniqueness*: The uniqueness of each client is recognized in WCT where personal truth and worth are seen as inseparable. The combination of the two realities allows for differentiation of the client that is not limited by the requirements in a system. The

unfolding of the process the client uses to develop a pattern of realized self-worth overtime increases the incomparableness of each person.

Truth: The client's honest self-evaluation will never diminish their BSW because their worth continues to exist even when a client is not aligned with it. To know and tell the truth about self to self is a valued practice for clients in WCT because they will come back into connection with the truth that BSW exists for them. Rogers and Stevens (1967) proposed that living one's truth is helpful as we move through life. Becoming more conscious of self without BSW can make a client more self-conscious, which can lead to suffering.

Self-sufficiency: A client can engage in environment-transcending patterns, which include building the four pillars of worth based on their recovered understanding of BSW. Myers and Sweeney (2004) suggested that coping effectively with the challenges of life increases a sense of worthiness in the individual. In WCT, this wellness value is present in the idea of a client migrating from the quadrant where they were born (i.e., Q1, Q2, or Q3) toward Q4 where self-worth is affirmed consistently.

Meaningfulness: The client can acknowledge and gain a deeper conscious recognition that human worth has a significant purpose in the lived experience of every person. A client who is looking for the will-to-meaning can look to what they value (Frankl, 1962) and discover that an inherent core value, BSW, is helpful in that endeavor. Furthermore, a life built on the foundation of BSW can better endure the senseless moves against self and humanity and still be meaningful, and thereby help to avoid the existential apathy vacuum that Viktor Frankl warned us about.

Worth-Conscious

In Chapter 2, we introduced Julian Jaynes' theory of consciousness and described how WCT aligns with his idea that humans are conscious beings. We support and use mindful processes, such as those used in acceptance and commitment therapy which help clients notice what thoughts play out in their mind without attributing either a positive or a negative label to those thoughts. One common idea in mindfulness is that people are taught to recognize their thoughts and the good or bad labels they attach to them. Being conscious of one's thoughts and the labels attached creates a novel point of view whereby the person can be both the actor and the audience of the experience that plays out on their mental stage. As an example of an actor on their own mental stage, consider a scene in which the actor is sitting next to a stream observing their thoughts printed on leaves that are floating by (Harris, 2019). While observing themself onstage and withholding the judgments that used to accompany some of those thoughts and allowing them to float unburdened downstream and out of view, the client is both acting out the scene and seeing the scene acted out (this second position, as audience, is more removed from the action).

In WCT, we consider that consciousness can come from being mindful, but that it is not simply a mindful exercise. Consciousness is something a client can develop and appreciate as awareness of awareness that can be noticed and directed. What is happening on the mental stage can be seen, experienced, and overseen. The client is the actor (i.e., their thoughts are represented on the mental stage), the audience (i.e., an observer of what happens on the mental stage), and the director (i.e., awareness of what could happen on the mental stage that may benefit the person in real life). The capacity to understand that BSW creates equity between any two worthy people when that reality has not been experienced may require some mental stage-directing skills. In other words, if our client is acting out an old pattern of denied self-worth in their mind, that denial shows up as a combination of thinking and feeling that was scripted. As the actor of that scene, our client is handed their system's well-used script, and they habitually start using the same set of thoughts and feelings required to play the scene in an old and acceptable way. Subsequently, when the scene is finished, feelings of worth are not experienced.

WCT clients can become more aware of their mental scene and can learn to observe the scene without judgment of either good or bad. However, observation in and of itself will not make clients feel more worthy. Although clients who are less self-critical/judgmental (i.e., attaching negative emotion to thoughts) may feel a reduction in anxiety, they will not likely experience a renewed sense of self-worth without an intentional focus on their BSW. Clients who have routinely had their self-worth needs denied may come to experience their self-worth needs as a burden and thereby fail to regard their needs as useful in developing a healthy sense of self. As such, WCT psychotherapists allow their clients' self-worth needs to be seen, respected, and esteemed so that clients can eventually gain the confidence needed to value and meet those needs themselves.

The psychotherapist will be worth-conscious and hold their clients' BSW in mind throughout the session(s). This means the psychotherapist is aware of a type of worthiness that clients cannot lose and understands that the client's worthiness may have been denied as a result of acquired values and conditions in the client's system. This initial awareness of BSW, which is consistent in the therapeutic process, sets the stage for the psychotherapist and client to collaboratively affirm client self-worth through the counseling experience. Another aspect of being worth-conscious as a helping professional is to provide unadulterated respect as the client shares their story. The story shared by the client may involve a problem that is considered easier to manage because it does not attach to the client's sense of self or worth. Even when a client is unable to express their lost-worth story, it is imperative that the psychotherapist conveys and models the importance of being worth-conscious throughout the counseling process. Unadulterated respect means that the psychotherapist protects and affirms the BSW of their client even when the client denies it or has accepted the denial of their BSW by others. In Chapter 7 of the Migrating to Q4 section, we discuss how psychotherapists can accomplish the task of protecting and affirming their clients' BSW.

The client is invited to provide feedback relevant to feeling respected by the psychotherapist and the counseling process. The client can also freely give their opinion about what they like and do not like about the experience with the option of vetoing an idea that the psychotherapist has that does not fit their sense of self. The first goal of the psychotherapist is to create an environment that fully recognizes the client's truth and worth and provides opportunity for the client to participate in co-creating and maintaining a safe and worth-affirming space where something therapeutic (either worth-based or not) can happen. This may be an unfamiliar experience for the client as they may assume that the worth-affirming experience is specific to being with a helping professional in a structured process.

As helping professionals, it is our responsibility to be especially careful so as not to repeat any aspect of denying our clients' worth in a familiar way. The stage we set in our counseling sessions will eventually become part of the mental stage of each client. As WCT psychotherapists, we introduce the basic concepts of WCT in all interactions with clients, even if they themselves have not yet established a pattern of affirming their BSW.

Self-Conscious

Duval and Wicklund's (1972) theory of objective self-awareness stated that human consciousness can be focused internally on the self or on external objects. In their theory, attention can be focused through awareness of self *onto self* (i.e., an awareness of self that is intentionally conscious of the thoughts and feelings one is experiencing) or shifted externally where the experience of being a social object can cause anxiety. They proposed that self-awareness can morph into self-consciousness, especially when the external focus on how a person appears to others can become problematic (i.e., anxiety-provoking). Although being self-conscious can be a good or bad experience in Duval and Wickland's theory, in WCT, it reflects an absence of being worth-conscious. We acknowledge that a person can suspend self-evaluation or judgment and be just conscious (i.e., neutral thinking) or conscientious (i.e., thoughtful about others). Self-consciousness is labeled with two possible types: private self-consciousness (internal reflection) and public self-consciousness (external effect). An internal focus enables self-evaluation which can allow a person to compare self in relation to a set of standards. The comparison of one's sense of self with standards can promote behavior change, which may support a feeling of pride but could also result in dissatisfaction. In WCT theory, we recognize self-consciousness as an internally held frame of reference that can be influenced by both private and public events, which have a negative effect on the person. In a self-conscious state of mind, a client can feel angst about being unworthy. Angst can develop into a more severe level of anxiety that is fear-based when the client is afraid of not measuring up or being compared to some introduced standard. Severe anxiety runs the risk of becoming pathological and can manifest as insecurities, over-striving, comparison driven anger, hopeless-ness and so forth.

Ingram (1990) stated that excessive self-focused attention or self-absorption was involved in the pathogenesis of multiple mental disorders. Among the specific mental health challenges are social anxiety, poor social performance, and negative self-judgments and attributions (Spurr & Stopa, 2002). In WCT, we consider self-consciousness to be an undesirable alternative to being worth-conscious. In the absence of having self-worth needs acknowledged and affirmed, clients will begin to construct a personal narrative using conditions. These conditions can include parental injunctions that allow clients to have an altered (non-worth-based) negative self-reference. The alteration in focus occurs when clients grow up having their life needs affirmed (e.g., food, shelter) and self-worth needs (e.g., awareness, respect, esteem of our BSW) denied, first by others and then by themselves as a matter of habit. When self-worth needs are not acknowledged and affirmed, they become easier for clients to ignore and deny, which can result in them questioning if their self-worth needs are useful or even real. The client's uncertainty surrounding the utility or realness of their self-worth needs can be understood as a lack of experience with having their needs honored in the system and a habitual pattern of their needs being ignored.

The WCT-trained psychotherapist will listen for their clients' words/narrative that inform their self-conscious feelings about being unacceptable within their system and within themselves. Several sessions may take place before a client reveals a sense of unworthiness. The psychotherapist will listen for signs of the client shifting into a self-conscious mental state, such as the client feeling desperate to make a good impression, or the client experiences anxiety about being judged by others. Yet another sign of self-consciousness is the client engaging in habitual self-doubt—never believing they are enough. Where a self-conscious frame of mind exists, the WCT psychotherapist will look for a possible culprit beneath that frame of reference, such as denied BSW.

We do not recommend moving quickly to name the possibility of denied self-worth; rather, we suggest that the psychotherapist follows the client's reason for seeking therapy and allows their client to create the pace of revealing any underlying fear about not being worthy.

Because fear can form in the absence of consistent affirmation of self-worth, the client's self-worth is transient or retractable. The client may have difficulty trusting their BSW if it has been denied. Even though the client's BSW was not always affirmed, it is still there waiting to be reaffirmed. Yet the client may find it easier to believe the denial they have experienced over the possibility of reaffirming their BSW. In a worst-case scenario, the client may feel hopeless and fully ensconced in the belief that they are doomed to live a life without feeling/being worthy. They may share part of their lost-worth story with trepidation because they are afraid that what they have experienced (denied BSW) is deserved or intractable.

Life Needs

Maslow (1968) created the hierarchy of needs which depicted the requirements for a firm foundation that provided support for achieving actualization. Actualization is when a person realizes their full potential. Maslow's theory proposes that humans are motivated to fulfill their needs in a hierarchical order, with the most basic needs being fulfilled before progressing to more advanced needs. Fulfilling one's full potential (i.e., actualization) can only be achieved after the basic needs of life are fulfilled. Maslow's basic life needs include physiological (e.g., food, water, clothing, warmth, rest), safety (e.g., shelter, security), and love and belonging (e.g., family, friends, intimate relationships). In WCT, when the basic life needs are not or cannot be met consistently within the family system, self-worth needs can still be honored but it is more difficult. We will discuss this challenge later in the section referencing Quadrant 2 and the life needs/self-worth needs diagram provided in Chapter 7.

Psychotherapists will informally assess, via a simple Q&A process, their clients' degree of fulfillment of basic life needs and assist them in obtaining the support they need. They will also discuss any gaps in the system for their clients who need support in fulfillment of their basic life needs and help them seek out alternatives. Compassionate honesty for the plight of clients in this situation (Quadrants 1 & 2) honors their BSW while educating them about available community resources, which helps get their basic needs met. In WCT, there is no shame in needing help with basic life needs.

Self-Worth Needs

According to the Jungian concept of individuation, the individuality of each person starts to take shape during infancy as the person begins to become who they are through self-discovery and eventually gain self-realization (Fordham, 1985). Acceptance of self as good enough (Stein, 2005) is eventually experienced through the process of individuation, which includes finding meaning in life. In WCT, self-worth is key in developing individuality, first as an affirmation of every infant having a birthright, a foundational privilege to just be, which includes being supported in their self-discovery (self-worth needs and life needs), and second to encourage the embodiment of BSW as a self-supporting life philosophy. The physiological needs (i.e., life needs) of the brain and body become obvious because the infant will coo or cry to signal those needs being met or unmet. The indetectable self-worth needs are also present as a secondary but vital experience that happens at the same time life needs are being met. When a parent picks up a crying baby to assess what is wrong, they can do so in an intentional and attentive manner, or they can display irritation, resentment, or apathy. In the case of the latter, the infant may start to pair having their life needs met with being unworthy of that experience.

When the earliest self-worth needs are recognized by caregivers and understood as connected to life needs, then the caregiver's conscientious attentiveness to life needs affirms self-worth needs (i.e., accepting the reality of the infant as existing and worthy). Similarly, and according to interpersonal neurobiology, children enjoy a nourishing relational experience when their caregiver responds to their basic needs with warm curiosity and delight (Badenoch, 2023). The quality of our early primary relationships shapes our expectations of what to anticipate when interacting with others, and some learn to expect nurturing. From a WCT perspective, nourishing includes life needs and self-worth needs being recognized and affirmed. The capacity to accept unconditionally an infant and how they are wired seems instinctual. The infant is signaling what they are experiencing, and those signals are respected as honest. WCT proposes that the same unconditional acceptance can continue throughout life when awareness of one's life and self-worth needs are respected as true for them. Physiological processes and the mental/emotional development of individuality during the earliest stages of childhood can be acknowledged, respected, and even esteemed by others. This affirmation of a person's truth and worth can be based on their experienced reality of signaling what they really need as they are being true to self and becoming more aware of who they are. Only that person knows what signals are going off in their brain and body and only they can communicate what that experience is like for them. People may not have labels for everything they are feeling, so others must listen and learn from them and exercise patience as people attempt to explain their experience and/or inherent values. The helper may not have the same inherent values and therefore lacks understanding of what others experience/value. Trusting the child's senses and signals and valuing what they are experiencing about themselves is vital to the development of the child's sense of self.

The psychotherapist will assess the extent to which the client recognizes their BSW. The presence of BSW means that some amount of self-worth needs has been met in the client's life. A lack of understanding of self as worthy does not mean that the client's self-worth needs were never met in childhood, but rather they were met inconsistently or conditionally, which made BSW appear transient. Once an adult client is seeking professional help, the psychotherapist starts to work backwards from the level of obtained BSW to determine how the client's self-worth needs were obtained or denied. To better understand the state of confusion (i.e., am I worthy or not?) and/or problems that the client presents with in session, the psychotherapist will work with the client to uncover the degree of BSW that was allowed in the system and denied in the client. An assessment of BSW as an integral sense of self includes listening to how the client was valued by others, and if their significance as a person was unconditional. The psychotherapist will also assess the ability of the client to live from their BSW by listening for when and how they do or do not. This includes listening for when the client moves against something they value or when the client allows others to move against something they value including any denial of their self-worth.

An assessment of the client's level of consciousness of BSW requires that the psychotherapist listen for and inquire about:

- What the client values and if self-worth is included as a core value.
- The level of awareness of self-worth in the system. This is where a client may state the conditions present in the system that when followed they felt some degree of worth or acceptance. A counterfeit to BSW may be present in the system that the client accepts as a required goal to achieve importance in the system.
- The level of respect for self-worth in the system. This is where a conversation about inherent values can begin.
- What was esteemed in the system, and what the client esteems about themself. This is where a conversation about acquired versus inherent values can begin.
- When and how the client feels confident (or not) in their self-worth. This is where a conversation about being true to self and remaining worthy is possible.
- A lost-worth story and how prevalent the practice of denying the self-worth of members in the family system has been, including conditions, requirements, expectations, and abuse that have made the client feel unworthy.

Due to the length of this chapter, we will present the concepts of realized self-worth and the lost-worth story in Chapter 5, and systemic exigencies and intrusive and abusive injunctions in Chapter 6. The descriptions of inherent and acquired values, as well as competing values, are embedded in the material in Chapter 3. The remaining content from the list of foundational concepts of WCT at the beginning of this chapter will be contained in Chapter 6 (i.e., Pillars) and Chapter 7 (i.e., Quadrants).

References

Badenoch, B. (2023). *The heart of trauma: Healing the embodied brain in the context of relationships*. New York, NY: Norton.

Crocker, J., Brook, A. T., Niiya, Y., & Villacorta, M. (2006). The pursuit of self-esteem: Contingencies of self-worth and self-regulation. *Journal of Personality*, 74(6), 1749–1772. https://doi.org/10.1111/j.1467-6494.2006.00427.x

Duval, S., & Wicklund, R. A. (1972). *A theory of objective awareness*. New York: Academic Press.

Fordham, M. (1985). *Explorations into the self*. The Library of Analytical Psychology. vol. 7, London: Academic Press.

Frankl, V. E. (1962). *Man's search for meaning: An introduction to logotherapy*. Boston: Beacon Press.

Friedrichs, J. (2016). An intercultural theory of international relations: How self-worth underlies politics among nations. *International Theory*, *8*(1), 63–96. https://doi.org/10/1017/S1752971915000202

Fukuyama, M. A., & Sevig, T. D. (1999). *Integrating spirituality into multicultural counseling*. (Vol. *13*). Thousand Oaks, CA: Sage Publications.

Harris, R. (2019). *ACT made simple: An easy-to-read primer on acceptance and commitment therapy*. Oakland, CA: New Harbinger Publications.

Ingram, R. E. (1990). Self-focused attention in clinical disorders: review and conceptual model. *Psychological Bulletin*, *107(2)*, 156–176. https://doi.org/10.1037/0033-2909.107.2.156

Maslow, A. H. (1968). *Toward a psychology of being*. (2nd ed.). New York, NY: D. Van Nostrand Company.

Myers, J. E., & Sweeney, T. J. (2004). The indivisible self: An evidence-based model of wellness. *Journal of Individual Psychology*, *60*(3), 234–245. https://core.ac.uk/download/pdf/149232976.pdf

Rogers, C. R., & Stevens, B. (1967). *Person to person: The problem of being human, a new trend in psychology*. Lafayette, CA: Real People Press.

Serrani, A. (2022). Joni Madraiwiwi Quotes That Remain Enriching. *Your Dictionary*, https://www.yourdictionary.com/articles/joni-madraiwiwi-enriching-quotes

Sevig, T. D., Highlen, P. S., & Adams, E. M. (2000). Development and validation of the Self-Identity Inventory (SII): A multicultural identity development instrument. *Cultural Diversity & Ethnic Minority Psychology*, *6*(2), 168–182. https://doi.org/10.1037/1099-9809.6.2.168

Shneidman, E. S. (1993). *Suicide as psychache: A clinical approach to self-destructive behavior*. Northvale, NJ/London: Jason Aronson.

Spurr, J. M. & Stopa, L. (2002). Self-focused attention in social phobia and social anxiety. *Clinical Psychology Review*, *22*, 947–975. https://doi.org/10.1016/s0272-7358(02)00107-1

Stein, M. (2005). Individuation: Inner Work. *Journal of Jungian Theory and Practice*, *7*(2), 1–13.

Svedberg, P., Hallsten, L., Narusyte, J., Bodin, L., & Blom, V. (2016). Genetic and environmental influences on the association between performance-based self-esteem and exhaustion: A study of the self-worth notion of burnout. *Scandinavian Journal of Psychology*, *57*(5), 419–426. http://doi.org/10.1111/sjop.12309

5

REALIZED SELF-WORTH, LOST-WORTH STORY, AND TRAUMA-INFORMED CARE

Realized Self-Worth

A belief sometimes called the democratic ideal was a common assumption across virtually all humanistic approaches (Grummon, 1965). The ideal can be summed up as the belief in the worth and dignity of each individual. Theorists such as Abraham Maslow, Carl Rogers, and Fritz Perls adopted this major assumption within the philosophy of humanism, which supports the belief that humans, as unique individuals, have a right and responsibility to be self-directing in their independence (Grummon, 1965). Rogers (1959) viewed the ability of human beings to be self-actualizing as one of the fundamental characteristics of all life, calling it the actualizing tendency. Self-actualization, as defined by Maslow (1968, p. 25), is the "ongoing actualization of potentials, capacities and talents, as fulfillment of mission (or call, fate, destiny, or vocation), as a fuller knowledge of and acceptance of, the person's own intrinsic nature, as an unceasing trend toward unity, integration, or synergy with the person."

Realized self-worth (RSW) is the practice and outcome of affirming birthright self-worth (BSW). In worth-conscious theory (WCT), a client can develop RSW in a natural way as part of a worth-affirming family system or a client can discover the benefits of RSW through their purposeful pursuit of becoming worth-conscious. WCT psychotherapists

 DOI: 10.4324/9781003599739-5

focus on the client's consciousness of self as worthy and the ramifications of believing self to be unworthy or less than worthy. We regard the realization of self-worth as a process that cannot be entered into without the client first experiencing BSW. The experience of having BSW can begin in the first year of life, but it does not have to. The attachment researcher and psychologist John Bowlby demonstrated through his research that children who experienced a secure attachment relationship with their parents felt protected, safe and worthy of love, which allowed them to explore their world more confidently (Bowlby, 1969). He also noted that a feeling of unworthiness and pervasive insecurity resulted from a lack of healthy attachment during childhood causing long-term emotional distress, which he referred to as insecure attachment styles. An insecure attachment style will impede the successful practice of realizing self-worth. We believe it is important to understand the basics of a lack of healthy attachment in order to see how it affects self-worth. Insecure attachment styles can arise from interactions with caregivers who are inconsistent and inadequate, which Bowlby described as anxious-ambivalent, avoidant, or disorganized. Individuals who are characteristic of an anxious-ambivalent attachment style display anxiety and uncertainty. They typically experienced caregivers who were inconsistent in their responses such that they may have been nurturing and responsive at times and neglectful and intrusive on other occasions. An avoidant attachment style is characterized by persons who may avoid closeness or intimacy and try not to rely on others or have others rely on them. This type of style stems from caregivers who were emotionally unavailable or unresponsive, resulting in one's preference for independence over connection. A disorganized attachment style is characterized by confusion and/or fear of not being worthy or deserving of love or emotional connectedness. Persons with this attachment style may display confusion because their caregivers were a source of both comfort and fear (i.e., unpredictable), much like what is seen in abuse and trauma scenarios (i.e., post traumatic stress disorder; PTSD).

Clients who have experienced an insecure attachment may be unaware of the impact that their style of attachment has had on their interpersonal relationships and their well-being. The lack of awareness can include a pre-conscious schema (i.e., outside of awareness), which is an automated protective reaction to a perceived threat that limits a client's conscious response in new situations. Attachment schemas form early in life and then predict future reactions in new exchanges with others within hundreds of milliseconds (Cozolino, 2010), like a watch-guard in a high tower of the mind. An attachment schema can be based on early experiences of safety, danger, or both. The implicit nature of a schema means that it can be unconscious and, therefore, that it shapes the potential conscious experiencing of others before our ability to perceive the truth or worth of the interaction is available. Stress can cause an insecure or disorganized schema to surface and set off a chain of internal events whereby embodied trauma (i.e., the physical manifestation of traumatic experiences) triggers a client's rapid approach-avoidance reaction to a perceived threat. This triggered reaction will preclude the client from feeling worthy and impede the practice of realizing self-worth because the client must endure the unconscious intrusion and then manage the aftershock over and over, which can leave them feeling ashamed. The trigger operates like a program that is designed for maximum protection, which disallows a conscious presence to first test for safety in others. In WCT, introducing the idea of a worth-conscious orientation to a client who does not have a secure attachment schema requires that the psychotherapist be mindful of the possibility that their client's experiences may be outside of conscious thought. The client may not believe that they can test the safety of new interactions because their watch-guard schema pulls up the draw bridge and shuts the gates. Psychotherapists should focus on introducing worth-conscious ideology slowly and reaffirm safety as they work to affirm their client's BSW. This purposeful reprogramming of the autonomic nervous system allows the client to recognize self-worth and personal truth as having always existed within them while also staying safe, and consistently holding onto this realization regardless of who moves to challenge their right to feel worthy and remain safe. Safety in the system allows for RSW to be pursued.

Raising client consciousness or 'conscientization' is the name of a consciousness-raising exercise that psychiatrist Pamela Seator enjoyed learning while working with the Peace Corps in Honduras in the mid-1970s. She had traveled with a Honduran colleague to small villages to engage the campesino women (i.e., women who supported the men who worked the land, typically on small plots, and who held a sense of belonging to the land) in conscientization activities. One particular activity that she recounted instructed the women to draw a circle on a piece of paper and include within the circle the important things in their village. Seator stated that what was striking to her was that these women placed the men, children, and chickens inside the circle but placed themselves outside the circle (personal communication, October 4, 2024). Due to their position in the community, the campesino women felt less valuable than the chickens in that system, and this activity may have been the first time many of them could see the oppressive dynamic.

In WCT, we invite psychotherapists to focus on helping clients expand their conscious thought without triggering a maladaptive stress response. This careful approach to introducing conscious thought can come from an already available worldview that is outside of the client's experience. As an example of a worldview encounter that raises conscious thought, we return to the above example of the Peace Corps volunteer who engaged directly with local communities. In this cross-cultural interaction, mutual understanding and dignity were promoted as the volunteer became consciously aware of the poverty and inequalities of these local communities. Sharing stories with our clients about the challenges and unfairness that others have experienced (e.g., Peace Corps story) may help to raise clients' personal consciousness (i.e., subjective awareness of oneself and surrounding systems with new provisional options) in a less-threatening context. In other words, a client who hears a story that is not directly related to them may find it easier/safer to explore a possible connection to the story (e.g., existing outside the circle) and their own challenges and life circumstances. More precisely, the Peace Corps story about existing outside the circle could resonate with a client who has felt excluded or marginalized in their family and/or larger systems. Stories can be a client's first understanding of a lack of realized self-worth in others that resonates with them; thereby, increasing consciousness about their worth in a small way.

Raising conscious thought can also come from the client's early family life memories when worth was affirmed without conditions. This option for raising consciousness draws from life stories the client is already comfortable with and can re-experience without being triggered. The psychotherapist can direct the client's attention to themselves in the system and open the discussion to looking for any circles that created exclusion of any family members, for any reason. When consciousness is experienced without traumatic recollection and is also maintained, clients can use this increased awareness to develop a worth-affirming practice. This worth-affirming practice provides the footing that is needed for clients to continue to extend their mental reach to include self-worth in conscious decision-making about the many aspects of their lives, which sets them up to become worth-conscious and to begin a pattern of realizing self-worth.

The process of realizing personal worth builds on the knowledge of one's BSW through a consistent conscious effort to honor oneself as worthy by engaging in purposeful action. RSW is therefore a prospect, practice, and pattern all individuals can engage to affirm self-worth daily. Building with worth-affirming blocks, which affirm self-worth through all stages of life, starts out as something to perceive before the prospect can become a practice. The perception of self-worth will begin during the earliest years of life for some children as their needs are worthy of notice and nurture. A client may perceive that they feel unworthy of having some of their needs met as a reason to begin psychotherapy. They may be unfamiliar with another individual (e.g., the psychotherapist) providing feedback in a kind and nurturing way, but this introduction to being treated as worthy (of being seen, heard, understood) can open perception to their BSW. The prospect includes the capacity of children and clients to assess and address their own self-worth needs to the point of building on the foundation of BSW. The capacity to feel worthy is bolstered by having both self-worth and life needs met in childhood, and talking through what was and was not available to the client in their childhood is a start to reaffirming that they deserved to have both sets of needs met.

RSW refers to the ability of a person to increase their worth-consciousness and understand their BSW as real and available. If a client's BSW was denied by members of their family of origin, participating in psychotherapy can provide a safe space where better building blocks are available. The practice component of RSW involves the client addressing their self-worth needs and using the new worth-affirming building blocks presented to them in session (although they can bring worth-affirming building blocks with them from any interaction that did not deny their self-worth). These building blocks, which are informed by

BSW, are moments of self-awareness, self-respect, self-esteem, and self-confidence that are shared in session with clients to have and use in their efforts to be worth-conscious both in and out of the therapeutic process. Once a client has a basic understanding of BSW and can experience the dignifying impact and understanding it creates, they can recognize the value of using worth-affirming building blocks in creating a wellness-oriented pattern. The pattern component of RSW is about creating a life theme grounded in personal worth that does not allow conditions, counterfeits, injunctions, or competing values to alter personal knowledge of one's truth and acceptability.

Clients who have a working understanding of BSW and value gaining RSW are well-positioned to confront each challenging situation they share in psychotherapy through a worth-conscious lens. The worth-affirming building blocks that are needed in any situation can be found and shared in psychotherapy as part of the practice of building the pillars of self-worth while also deepening the realization process. There are many therapeutic techniques available through established psychotherapies which can help a client experience BSW and establish a practice of realizing self-worth as a lifelong affirmer. We will share some psychological techniques that have been modified to support WCT or that can be employed to affirm self-worth in Chapter 8.

Lost-Worth Story

The lost-worth story (LWS) begins during our earliest years of learning about ourselves. It is the experience of denied self-worth by one member against another during childhood and can last a lifetime. Our sense of self is rooted in the original conceptualization and communications about us that colored our earliest life experiences. Child psychologist Haim Ginott championed mutually respectful dialogue between caregivers and their children and directed parents to provide sane messages to their children because parental statements affect a child's self-worth (Ginott, 1972). He argued against parental messages that cause a child to distrust their own perception, disown their feelings, or doubt their worth. He further suggested that during childhood, doubting one's self-worth can begin with language such as blaming, shaming, preaching, moralizing, bossing, accusing, ridiculing, belittling, bribing, and threatening, which can determine one's destiny. The experience of not being seen, heard, felt, or understood as having basic human worth can deny the development of a worth-affirming narrative. Ginott's assertion that early relational history becomes implicitly embodied and will whisper subjective truth that shapes one's self-perception is consistent with an interpersonal neurobiology (IPNB) perspective. In other words, a client's experience of unworthiness from a relational pattern of denied self-worth, like all implicit memory, goes quickly and deeply into their long-term mental/emotional storage (Ecker, Ticic, Hulley, 2012), where the idea of being unworthy or conditionally worthy can replace their BSW. When our self-worth needs are not met, we can make up or adopt a story about why we did not deserve to have our self-worth needs acknowledged or affirmed. The denial of self-worth from birth through our formative years may allow the LWS to take root before we are fully conscious of ourselves.

According to Antonio Damasio, consciousness begins when we experience "wordless knowledge" that is at first a felt new knowledge, which leaves an impression on us that we call, *Me* (Damasio, 1999, p. 26). Consciousness is an experience where simultaneously we are seeing, smelling, hearing, touching, and tasting as we engage in interactions with others (and the world) and name those events as happening to me, whereas other organisms refer to these same stimuli as there or then— not as me being aware of me receiving stimulus and making a mental image (Damasio, 1999). The roots of an individual's LWS can and do feel as old as the individual themself if the mental images they hold about 'self' include worth-denying messages. Denied self-worth can come in many forms. In WCT, we name several ways that individual worth can be denied in childhood: conditions on BSW, counterfeits to RSW, abusive injunctions (e.g., shaming, verbal, and/or emotional cruelty), or intrusive injunctions (e.g., requiring the adoption of acquired values over embracing inherent values). The conditions of worth in family systems caused some clients to take their eye off BSW and focus attention on something acceptable in the system. Conditions gave family members something else to focus on that was allowed (or celebrated) in the system but did not increase worthiness. Counterfeits in the system silently oppose the development of RSW by promoting a systemic goal based on some of the acceptable conditions. Family members in the system gain a limited type of acceptability for upholding the family goal/dream that is based on conditions. Injunctions were the rules that created conformity and clients who were controlled by mental, emotional, physical, or spiritual injunctions may have internalized the communication within the experience of conforming. This internalized communication about not being good enough to exist without conforming in some way becomes the language of a LWS. An additional source of a LWS may come from parents (or influential people) who are living their own LWS. Consequently, a client may have learned and borrowed language from influential others that informs their life script, a story intrenched in a pattern of behavior which inhibits spontaneity and flexibility (Berne, 1964), and that reinforces a worth-denying narrative. We use the concept of a life script here to connote an overall story that can encase a LWS and include intergenerational losses from larger systemic experiences that made denying worth as an individual possible.

Repeating the LWS language as part of an internal dialogue unintentionally reinforces the denial of BSW. A client may start looking for evidence that they are not deserving of having their self-worth needs met; sadly, if worth is lost, all is lost. Self-worth needs that are consistently unmet can lead to a hardening or abandoning of self, which is hurtful and potentially damaging to one's well-being. That hurtful experience repeated throughout years of living (being worthy and not being treated as worthy) is confusing, frustrating, and eventually demoralizing. The outcome of creating a LWS is that the communication of being unworthy starts out in moments as words, these become actions, and actions can turn into habits. Habits that are practiced long enough become a pattern of behavior, which can feel inescapable. Clients who accept themselves as unworthy of essential human needs and who repeat this pattern of unworthiness until it is an entrenched way of life are condemned to a life that is alienated from their truth.

The impact severity of a LWS story on a client's well-being varies from individual to individual. A less problematic pattern of denied self-worth would mean that a client had some of their self-worth needs met consistently for a period of time in their development and that they were able to build some or all of the pillars of self-worth (i.e., awareness, respect, esteem, confidence) to some degree. The more fully constructed their pillars of self-worth, the lower the practice of denying BSW and therefore the less doubt of having human worth. The less constructed the four pillars of self-worth are, the more fearful the client may feel about potentially losing worthiness or having lost it and having to pretend that it exists. The most severe story of lost worth is traumatizing and can retraumatize a client with each retelling. This most severe level of denied BSW is evidence of unconstructed pillars of self-worth, rejected inherent values, and internalized abusive injunctions—allowing the individual to distrust the existence of BSW as real for them (or anyone).

From a clinical perspective, we propose the terms listed in Figure 5.1 to capture the levels of disrupted well-being that a client can experience when a LWS is present and or repeated. There are certainly more experiences that can be included amongst the terms we have identified to reflect the varied levels of disrupted well-being. As such, we encourage psychotherapists to work with their clients to identify those experiences and to decide where their description of lost worthiness is best represented on the proposed diagram. The psychotherapist can show the chart to clients and ask them where on the chart the disruptive experience belongs (for them). If the client is at the self-doubt level, the psychotherapist can ascertain what degree of doubt is occurring. Is the client doubting that a particular person they interact with sees them as unworthy, or are they doubting their own worth? If they are doubting their worthiness, is it situational (one incident—a few incidents) or is it pervasive (the doubt is contaminating other interactions and becoming a habit of thought)?

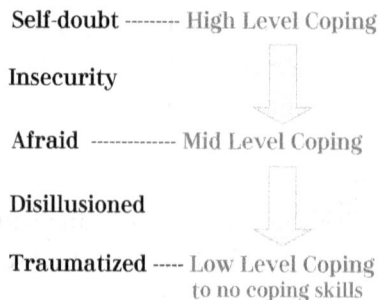

Self-doubt -------- High Level Coping

Insecurity

Afraid ------------ Mid Level Coping

Disillusioned

Traumatized ----- Low Level Coping
to no coping skills

Figure 5.1 Disrupted Well-Being and Coping.

The gateway to insecurity is a pervasive type of doubt that can be indicative of a habit of doubting self-worth. Psychotherapists are encouraged to explore with their client how doubting their self-worth has affected their insecurity. The next category on the chart, Insecurity, embodies self-doubt about having BSW to the extent that it shifts the inner reality of the client away from trusting that their BSW exists, thereby reducing their self-confidence. Because the level of disruption marked by client insecurity involves more pervasive self-doubt, external events that may or may not be directed toward the client can pass through a disruptive mental filter and allow the client to misinterpret the words and actions of others as confirmation that they lack BSW. Being insecure about having or deserving BSW can be situational within certain systems or with certain people who consistently treat them as if their worth means nothing; thereby, widening the gap (i.e., where BSW is erased) by negatively impacting both self-confidence and self-esteem.

When the client has enough experience with people who treat their worth as nothing special, they may become afraid that the gap is truer than having a birthright that dignifies their existence. Afraid, as a level of disruption, includes self-doubt and insecurity about basic human worth and adds the internal dimension of a habit of mind that can shift the client into a state of fearfulness. A state of fearfulness can be practiced to the point that it becomes a pattern of behavior marked by low self-confidence and lessening self-esteem as the client dislikes the fear-based version of themself. Once that pattern has been implemented through perpetual fear-based thinking, disillusionment can set in. At this point, BSW has become illusive, giving rise to a disillusioned state of mind that feels inescapable. Clients find that their coping skills are ineffective against the possibility that BSW is unavailable to them in most of their interactions. Consequently, the gap that BSW could have sealed has grown (through worth-denying messaging) and is now filled with experiences representing a fight for significance that they cannot win alone. The experience of disruption, which includes low self-confidence, low self-esteem, and a lessening of/to low self-respect, is just one step away from an overall sense of trauma because the fear that we are nothing to most people has been reinforced to the point where it is personally distressing and disturbing.

Whereas high-level coping coincides with stressful experiences that still allow capacity to affirm self as worthy (e.g., self-doubt), low-level coping coincides with stressful experiences that disallow the ability or interest to affirm self as worthy (e.g., traumatized). Social and psychological stressors that culminate into fatalistic despair (hopelessness) and serious self-devaluation (helplessness) can severely challenge a person's ability to cope (Klott, 2012). Both helplessness and hopelessness as personally debilitating psychological pain fall under the traumatized level of disrupted well-being. Feelings of hopelessness and helplessness are hallmarks of psychache, which lead to a pervasive pattern of disbelief and/or denial about one's personal worth. Over time, this perpetual denial of self-worth negatively impacts all four pillars of self-worth. Awareness of self as worthy is the last of the four pillars to be affected by the LWS. The diminishment of awareness of self along with the lessening of the other three pillars (i.e., respect, esteem, confidence) contribute to feelings of hopelessness and helplessness. The goal of assessing clients' degree of disrupted well-being is threefold: (a) to identify coping skills that help them to manage the conditions, injunctions, and competing values that they are contending with; (b) to honor coping skills that affirm self-worth and introduce BSW-affirming skills from WCT; and (c) to co-assess with the client the severity of their denied BSW that required the current coping strategies. Consistent with a WCT perspective, we invite psychotherapists to pursue trauma-informed training so that they are skillfully prepared to support clients who present with a trauma level of disrupted well-being. Trauma-informed care has specific guidelines such that, when followed, the client is not retraumatized during the course of seeking understanding of self, and how self-worth was erased over time through a process of denying it both personally and systemically.

The ability to cope with systemic stressors is beneficial. Moreover, if a client demonstrates some level of coping, they are communicating that there is indeed something worth coping for. Although coping skills that have helped clients feel a sense of worthiness can be viewed as useful, those skills may need to be modified to reflect a proactive mindset rather than a reactive one. Clients can proactively hold their BSW in a place of significance mentally and emotionally or they can be unsure of having

BSW, not consciously hold it, and therefore fight with others and themselves to believe it exists for them. A reactive mindset is indicative of a client feeling unworthy in an interaction with someone and fighting to hold onto their value during and after the incident. The client may hold the words or the actions of the worth-denying event in their mind as evidence that BSW does not exist for them and use energy to counter the disruptive messaging. Woefully, the energy a client expends to fight the disruptive messaging is immense and could instead be used to be themselves. Clients may say things to themselves such as, "I am okay," on repeat but not feel okay. The gap created when BSW is not affirmed becomes the experience that clients are most afraid of because they fear it is more real than their human worth. The equation (BSW + a series of events negating BSW = doubt and eventually despair) may be simplified in the mind of a client: if I was really worthy, the gap would not exist. A gap of doubt that can foster insecurity and evolve into disillusionment provides evidence that a feeling of nothingness can replace something as significant as the human worth within us.

Recognizing Trauma

Not all traumatic events have a detrimental impact on BSW; however, both one-time events and multiple smaller events can traumatize a client and make them feel unworthy. The accumulation of multiple (think hundreds to millions) small worth-denying infractions may cause a similar severity of biological and psychological symptoms seen in survivors of major traumatic events. Developmental trauma in childhood is caused by exposure to a variety of multiple invasive traumatic events, of an interpersonal nature (mo.gov, 2023). In his book *The Trauma of Everyday Life*, Mark Epstein, psychiatrist and author, wrote about the need for psychotherapists to understand the impact of developmental trauma on clients. He wanted psychotherapists to tie their understanding of a certain mental state he named, ascetic strain in the contemporary psyche, to something deeper in the client's developmental history. Epstein interpreted the parent–child relationship as the basis for meeting or failing to meet the infant's ruthless needs of appetite and distress. Parents either try to make those earliest needs bearable and succeed, or do not adequately manage the intensity of the needs of their child and their child is left with overwhelming emotions that they are ill-equipped to handle alone. These distressing emotions about unmet needs can eventually "turn into self-hate" (Epstein, 2013, p. 23), which a client subsequently experiences as anxiety or depression.

Complex post-traumatic stress disorder (C-PTSD) is a type of trauma in adults resulting from developmental trauma in childhood. Clients experiencing C-PTSD were likely children who grew up in a family that ignited their defense mechanisms so often that they developed a pattern of fight, flight, freeze, or fawn that was quickly triggered and difficult to decommission (Walker, 2013). In WCT, we believe that a LWS develops because self-worth needs were not adequately met. When clients' self-worth needs are consistently unmet and their coping skills fail to help them manage the unworthiness that was fostered in their system, psych-ache (i.e., psychological pain) develops which, in turn, leads to trauma. In other words, clients who have felt helpless with getting their needs met, and who have been unsuccessful with communicating their needs to their caregivers, may experience hopelessness. We contend that the hopeless-ness is due to ineffective coping mechanisms that have left clients feeling unworthy and exhausted from needing something reinforced that contin-ues to be denied by systems and self.

Clients who experience a combined state of helplessness and hopeless-ness may be exhausted from contending with the symptoms of prolonged trauma. Not being able to get above the struggle, personally or systemi-cally, contributes to this potentially deadly duo of disempowerment. The beleaguered client is burdened with a combination of symptoms resulting from repeated trauma, which can include mental, emotional, and physi-cal expression and associated features such as dissociation, hyperarousal, hypo-arousal, self-recrimination, shattered assumptions, mood distur-bances, addictions, impulsive behaviors, somatic complaints, overcom-pensations, repetition compulsion, self-harm, or other self-destructive behavior. Symptoms might also manifest as alexithymia (i.e., the inability to recognize or describe one's own emotions) and/or changes in person-ality (Schiraldi, 1999). To add to the struggle, clients may personalize the injustice and suffer moral injury. Judith Herman (1997) listed altera-tions in affect regulation, consciousness, self-perception, perception of perpetrator, relations with others, and systems of meaning as common in clients suffering from C-PTSD.

It is important to note that trauma can be the result of limited or one-time exposure to an event that does not increase a sense of unworthiness. In response to a unique traumatic event, Forcén (2021) wrote about a case of cinematic neurosis (i.e., trauma from watching a film) that occurred in Kansas during the summer of 1975, in which a 17-year-old girl was admitted to Wesley Medical Center in Wichita for nuchal rigidity, jerking of the limbs, and hallucinations of being attacked by sharks. After a thorough workup, the doctors concluded that the patient had a psychological rather than a biological issue. The patient would engage in episodic screaming calling out, "Sharks! Sharks!" while jerking her limbs in agitation. Dr. Forcén (2021) clarified that it was out of the ordinary for a girl who lived in Kansas, thousands of miles from the ocean, to suffer somatic manifestations from a fear of sharks. He explained that the girl from Kansas admitted that she had recently watched the film *Jaws*. Her psychological trauma happened from an imagined threat that was a sizeable one-time event to cause severe anxiety. After discharge, the case was written up by her neurologist and published in the *New England Journal of Medicine*. Although the girl's trauma was based on fear provoked by exposure to images that she was not mentally or emotionally prepared to handle, it most likely did not impact her self-worth. It is the readiness or ability to handle worth-denying messages that we are most concerned with. Nevertheless, we wanted to provide readers with a trauma event that affected coping skills but not BSW. Fear-based thinking can show up in many ways, including fear for physical safety, but one of the imperceptible ways fear-based thinking can progress into C-PTSD involves the slow death of BSW by a million cuts.

Trauma occurs when a client's resiliency and resources fail to support their well-being. To clarify further, a client's coping skills stop affirming the existence of an elusive self-worth and then messaging that denies BSW overflows into their mind and heart, flooding consciousness. The client's LWS is indicative of some degree of denied BSW, the level of damage that is done to the four pillars of self-worth, and the pervasiveness of disruption to their well-being. Substantial damage to the four pillars of self-worth erodes the coping skills that are associated with those pillars, which can result in symptoms of C-PTSD as an adult. The most severe level of disrupted well-being diminishes resiliency and causes trauma for the client.

IPNB understandings of trauma emphasize that it can occur when we do not have the support needed to integrate a fearful or painful experience into the flow of our developing brain. Moreover, our embodied brains' capacity to receive worth affirmation in the form of physical/ mental/emotional nourishment can be shaped and diminished in powerful ways during our early years in the family system where trauma can become embedded (Badenoch, 2023). Without empathetic support or the necessary internal resources, a challenge or difficult circumstance can turn from potential trauma to embedded trauma. In contrast to a single traumatic event, embedded trauma refers to psychological wounds that are deeply ingrained and associated with long-standing experiences of distress, suffering, and emotional pain (e.g., abuse, neglect, violence, systemic oppression and so forth). Trauma-informed care is a therapeutic modality that should be considered when addressing these deep-rooted injuries.

Trauma-Informed Care

If the client presents with symptoms of helplessness and hopelessness it is critical to provide trauma-informed care or to refer the client to a clinician with such training. It goes without saying that a suicide assessment should be completed if the client's hopelessness is accompanied by suicidal ideation. Trauma-informed care is a specific mental health modality and mission developed by the Substance Abuse and Mental Health Services Administration, with principles and guidelines that support the national and international health and well-being of people and systems. They name three "E's" of trauma, stating that individual trauma results from a series of *events*, or set of circumstances, *experienced* as harmful (physically or emotionally) or life-threatening, that causes adverse *effects* to the well-being of the person's ability to function mentally, physically, socially, emotionally, or spiritually (Substance Abuse and Mental Health Services Administration, 2014).

WCT principles are in support of the three E's of trauma and remind us that, specific to the consistent undermining of BSW, a client can endure multiple *events* over years that move against their worth and subsequently their well-being. The *experience* of having BSW denied persistently by others is harmful to a client's overall sense of self. If the client adopts the pattern of denying self-worth, they can repeat traumatizing messaging and retraumatize themselves. The adverse *effect* of internalizing a pattern of denying BSW is best understood based on the degree of abdicated self-worth. The most severe outcome of surrendering one's BSW is the absence of experiencing self as real and worthy, which is counter to well-being.

To further understand how to assess a client's level of disruption that has elevated to the experience of trauma, we invite psychotherapists to enroll in on-line and/or in-person trauma workshops that are targeted to mental health providers, offered by reputable organizations and delivered by credentialed/licensed professionals. In WCT, we borrow a tool implemented by the San Francisco Department of Health (Kimberg & Wheeler, 2019) called the four C's of trauma-informed care (see Table 5.1), which provides guidance to clinicians who are working with clients who have symptoms of any type of trauma. If a psychotherapist is conducting a session in which the client's level of disruption is being assessed but their severity of trauma is unknown, especially if the psychotherapist has not yet gained the necessary trauma-informed training, we recommend applying the four C's of trauma-informed care.

The four C's emphasize principles of trauma-informed care and can serve mental health professionals as a touchstone to guide immediate and

Table 5.1 The Four C's of Trauma-Informed Care

Calm
- Pay attention to how you are feeling when you are caring for the patient. Breathe deeply and calm yourself to model and promote calmness for the patient, yourself, and your co-workers
- Practice calming exercises (deep breathing, grounding) with patients
- Cultivate understanding of trauma and its effects to promote a calm, patient attitude toward others (patients and co-workers)
- Re-design healthcare environments, policies, and practices to reduce chaos and promote calmness
- Cultivate understanding of how resilience, justice, and equity build peaceful, calm communities and environments

---

(Continued)

Table 5.1 (Continued)

Contain

— Limit trauma history detail to maintain emotional and physical safety. Provide education, resources, and referrals to trauma-specific care without requiring disclosure of trauma
— Model healthy relationship boundaries and earn trust by behaving reliably
— Monitor patients' emotional and physical responses to education and inquiry about trauma
— Practice calming techniques to help patient (or parent/caregiver and child dyad) regain composure
— Normalize fear of returning to the healthcare setting if the triggering of a trauma response occurs; invite the patient to share what changes would make visits more tolerable and healing
— Enact healthcare policies and practices that minimize re-traumatization of patients and staff
— Form multidisciplinary and multi-sector partnerships that reduce re-traumatization for patients and staff

Care

— Practice self-care and self-compassion while caring for others
— Share messages of support when patients disclose trauma or trauma symptoms
— Normalize and de-stigmatize trauma symptoms and harmful coping behaviors (as common sequelae of trauma)
— Practice cultural humility
— Adopt behaviors, practices, and policies that minimize and mitigate power differentials to reduce trauma and structural violence
— Enact healthcare policies that promote self-care, compassion, and equity
— Form equitable partnerships to extend CARE into the community

Cope

— Emphasize coping skills, positive relationships, and interventions that build resilience
— Inquire about practices that help the patient feel better and more hopeful
— Document a "Coping Strategies" list instead of only "Problem Lists" and include patient's own words of wisdom and good self-advice in the "after-visit" summary
— Improve identification and treatment of the mental health, substance use, and other sequelae of trauma
— Connect patients and families with community organizations to increase social support and access to necessary resources
— Promote equity within healthcare organizations, communities, and society

Source: Trauma and trauma-informed care. In M. R. Gerber (Ed.), *Trauma-informed healthcare approaches: A guide for primary care* (pp. 25–56), by L. Kimberg & M. Wheeler (2019). Springer. Adapted with permission. (see https://www.acesaware.org/wp-content/uploads/2019/12/Chapter-2-Trauma-and-Trauma-Informed-Care.pdf).

Table 5.2 Books on Trauma

Author	Title
Dana, Deb	*Polyvagal Theory in Therapy*
Fisher, Janina	*Healing the Fragmented Selves of Trauma Survivors: Overcoming Internal Self-alienation*
Herman, Judith	*Trauma and Recovery*
Mate, Gabor	*The Myth of Normal*
Ogden, Pat	*Trauma and the Body: A Sensorimotor Approach to Psychotherapy*
Porges, Stephen	*The Polyvagal Theory: Neurophysiological Foundations of Emotions, Attachment, Communication, and Self-regulation*
van der Kolk, Bessel	*The Body Keeps the Score: Brain, Mind, and Body in the Healing of Trauma*

sustained behavior change (Kimberg & Wheeler, 2019). WCT psychotherapists can assess the level of disrupted well-being in a client and realize during the process of assessment that a client has suffered trauma that requires a trauma-informed process. Whereas the lack of self-worth may still be a primary concern of the client, their need to feel safe enough to do self-worth specific psychotherapy may be best obtained via the psychotherapist's training in trauma-informed care. Following trauma-informed training, the psychotherapist can proceed to employ WCT concepts. When pursuing trauma training for the different types of trauma (i.e., shock, developmental, relational, and C-PTSD), psychotherapists can seek certification as a Certified Clinical Trauma Professional (CCTP). The list of books by trauma experts (see Table 5.2) provide a good foundation for understanding the development and impact of different types of trauma.

References

Badenoch, B. (2023). *The heart of trauma: Healing the embodied brain in the context of relationships*. New York, NY: Norton.

Berne, E. (1964). *Games people play*. New York: Ballantine Books.

Bowlby, J. (1969). Attachment and loss. Vol *1: Attachment. Basic Books*. New York.

Cozolino, L. (2010). *The neuroscience of psychotherapy: Healing the social brain*. New York, NY: Norton.

Damasio, A. R. (1999). *The feeling of what happens: Body and emotion in the making of consciousness.* New York: Mariner Books.

Ecker, B., Ticic, R., & Hulley, L. (2012). *Unlocking the emotional brain: Eliminating symptoms at their root using memory reconsolidation.* New York, NY: Routledge.

Epstein, M. (2013). *The trauma of everyday life.* New York: The Penguin Press.

Forcén, F. E. (2021). *Jaws and cinematic neurosis that persists. Psychiatric Times.* https://www.psychiatrictimes.com/view/jaws-and-cinematic-neurosis-that-persists

Ginott H. G. (1972). *Teacher and child: A book for parents and teachers.* New York: Macmillan.

Grummon, D. L. (1965). Client-centered theory. In B. Stefflre (Ed.), *Theories of counseling.* (pp. 30–90). New York: McGraw-Hill.

Herman J. L. (1997). *Trauma and recovery (Rev.).* New York: Basic Books.

Kimberg, L. & Wheeler, M. (2019). Trauma and trauma-informed care. In M. R. Gerber (Ed.), *Trauma-informed healthcare approaches: A guide for primary care.* (pp. 25–56). Springer.

Klott, J. (2012). *Suicide and psychological pain: Prevention that works.* Eau Claire, WI: PESI Publishing & Media.

Maslow, A. H. (1968). *Toward a psychology of being* (2nd ed.). New York: Van Nostrand Reinhold.

Mo.gov (2023). Missouri's early care and education connections. *Trauma-informed care.* https://earlyconnections.mo.gov/professionals/trauma-informed-care#

Rogers, C. R. (1959). A theory of therapy, personality, and interpersonal relationships, as developed in the client-centered framework. In S. Koch (Ed.), *Psychology: A study of science* (Vol. *III*). New York: McGraw-Hill.

Substance Abuse and Mental Health Services Administration. (2014). SAMHSA's Concept of Trauma and Guidance for a Trauma-Informed Approach. HHS Publication No. (SMA) 14-4884. Rockville, MD: Substance Abuse and Mental Health Services Administration.

Schiraldi, G. R. (1999). *The post-traumatic stress disorder sourcebook: A guide to healing, recovery, and growth.* New York: McGraw-Hill.

Walker, P. (2013). *Complex PTSD: From surviving to thriving.* Lafayette, CA: Azure Coyote.

6

SYSTEMIC EXIGENCIES AND THE FOUR PILLARS OF SELF-WORTH

Systemic Exigencies

A systemic requirement that denies personal truth and thereby obscures self-worth creates conformity to the demand at the expense of authenticity. Several types of exigencies are possible, but not all families employ the same rigid requirements for the same goals. In a family system, a goal to achieve can be grounded in the birthright self-worth (BSW) of each member or it can be fixed to a counterfeit (i.e., a false pretense that replaces the development of realized self-worth [RSW]) that sets the members up to lose their BSW in pursuit of the goal. This is not necessarily an explicit pattern known by the members with power in the system. The power they enjoy when they are enforcing systemic exigencies may have come with its own price; therefore, requiring adherence to a goal-defending but worth-denying practice may be commonplace. We will discuss the many possible counterfeits in the next section, but we mention the problem here because conformity with no reward does not compel an individual to be complicit in their own self-worth-denying practice. The reward in some systems for agreeing to the exigent rules is continued acceptance as a valued participant in pursuit of a goal upheld as more important than anything else or any single person. For example, power, success, or achieving a desired outcome is more important than

DOI: 10.4324/9781003599739-6

permission to be one's authentic self. A family or larger system with an attractive goal (e.g., wealth, status, superiority), even if it is a counterfeit to realizing individual BSW, can command or demand loyalty to the goal through the use of injunctions (i.e., direct statements and potent instructions about who the child/person must be that disallows their truth and worth). The client may have grown up assuming that allegiance to the family goal was necessary for enjoying continued acceptance as a member. They may not have considered that choosing a different path was possible, or they may have come to believe that another option was impossible. In some systems, choosing another way, other than the one that achieves the required goal (counterfeit), is criticized, judged, and ridiculed. In the cases where loyalty to the goal is demanded, the person wanting something different may be named as the problem through the use of a specific exigency, such as an intrusive or an abusive injunction. The level of severity of abuse through worth-denying injunctions is an important historical context in understanding the price a client has had to pay to remain acceptable in the system.

Transactional analysis as a psychoanalytic theory and method of psychotherapy (Berne, 1964) employed the idea of parental injunctions as an implicit way for parents to command or control the child. The child internalized the underlying message of the injunction and stayed stuck in the rhetoric. In consideration of transactional analysis, an older male psychotherapy client rejected any techniques which required him to parent himself by engaging in more responsible behavior. The psychotherapist was unsure why the rejection of only certain techniques was happening. In speaking with the client about those techniques that involved understanding the different ego states in transactional analysis (i.e., Parent, Adult, Child Ego states), the psychotherapist recognized the client's unwillingness to explore the advantages of parenting himself. He had always had his life needs met or exceeded, and he reported being financially stable for life. He let the psychotherapist know that he was not in psychotherapy to become a boring grown up; he was in psychotherapy because he just wanted somebody to talk to. He added the current challenge of not having very many friends, but having many weekly appointments with multiple professionals. The psychotherapist hypothesized that this client was following an old parental injunction, *Don't Grow Up*, among other challenges that involved an adult in perpetual child mode.

In WCT, the term injunction is derived from earlier theories, such as the work of Goulding and Mary (1978) who named twelve distinct injunctions: *Don't exist, Don't be important, Don't be you, Don't be a child, Don't grow up, Don't succeed, Don't be close, Don't belong, Don't think* (about something forbidden or differently from parents), *Don't feel* (a forbidden feeling or different feeling from parents), *Don't be well* (or Don't be sane), and *just Don't* (a command prohibiting of various activities). Parental injunctions are communicated from the parents' own "feelings of inadequacy, confusion, discontent, anxiety, unhappiness, disappointment, anger, frustration, and secret desires" (Budiša et al., 2012, p. 28). In WCT, we introduce two types of injunctions: intrusive and abusive. An intrusive injunction instructs the child to adhere to a condition of acceptability that coincidentally moves against their BSW. Instead of the derogatory message being abusive, like *Don't be you*, the intrusive message is more subtle with a condition that allows for importance or acceptance to be achieved such as, *Be the version of you that I like*. A young girl who was going outside to play with friends called out to her mom that she was leaving; her mom came to the top of the stairs and questioned her daughter, "Are you going out like that?" There was incrimination in her tone of voice. The 12-year-old looked down at her clothing and shrugged her shoulders, "Sure," she said quietly. She had been through this drill before, if she did not look good then her mom would not look good. She also knew that she only looked good enough if she looked the way her mom required—even to play kick-the-can in the neighborhood. The intrusion was not always overt, like being told to change her clothing and put on something better. She had been exposed to this maternal intrusion enough that just the act of questioning her before going was enough for her to feel wrong. A counterfeit in this system was to look good to others; it included conditions about acceptability that involved an intrusive injunction, *Only go out in public if I have approved how you look*.

To add to this story, if this parent used an abusive injunction, the child would not only be questioned, but also called names or reprimanded for not putting on the right (or best) clothing. This requirement can be both overtly and covertly communicated over a lifetime of outings and family get-togethers. The abusive injunction does not just invite conformity; it punishes nonadherence to conditions and non-pursuit of desirable counterfeits. The child is named as the problem and when their individuality gets in the way of achieving the desired outcome, they are shamed into submission with worth-denying messages and potential rejection or expulsion.

Table 6.1 provides a list of the original twelve parental injunctions used in transactional analysis and some of the corresponding WCT intrusive and abusive injunctions. Not all possible statements/messages can be listed because there are hundreds of iterations. The original twelve injunctions are listed in the first column as a point of reference for the different types of injunctions; however, we do not believe that there is a limit to the variety of injunctions possible in either of the WCT categories. We have listed items in the table that capture the tone of the different types of injunctions that deny BSW in either subtle or more harsh ways.

Table 6.1 Intrusive and Abusive Injunctions

Transactional Analysis	Intrusive and Abusive Injunctions in Worth-Conscious Theory	
Parental Injunctions	Intrusive Injunctions	Abusive Injunctions
Don't be a child.	Grow up, Be easier to be around.	I won't take care of you.
Don't grow up.	Stay innocent, Be my little baby.	I will fall apart if you change.
Don't succeed.	You're almost good enough.	You can't out-achieve me.
Don't be close.	Be less needy. Be stronger.	Get away, you bother me.
Don't belong.	You could fit in if you…	Nobody notices you.
Don't think.	Let me figure that out for you.	I do all the thinking for this family.
Don't feel.	Be less emotional.	Your feelings are irrelevant.
Don't be well.	I need you to need me.	You'll never make it on your own.
Don't exist.	Be smaller, Take up less space.	I wish you were never born.
Don't be important.	Boost my importance, Don't outshine me.	You'll never amount to anything.
Don't…	Any message that intrudes on the truth or worth in a subtler way.	Any overt or covert message that abuses sense of self-worth.

The psychotherapist will listen to which injunctions the client struggles with and will ask open-ended questions to learn more about the extent to which the injunctions continue to have an impact on the client's mental health. The client may feel guilty or ashamed to speak about the abuse and also find it challenging to speak ill of their parent. If the psychotherapist chimes in too soon with a statement validating the negative event(s), the client may perceive the psychotherapist as moving against their parent (something the client is struggling to not do) and thereby respond by defending their parent. In essence, the client may have chosen attachment over authenticity to stay acceptable in the family system, and any perception that the psychotherapist is moving against their parent could feel quite unsettling. The client may start to tell part of their story that includes the use of an injunction and then stop themselves from continuing because they feel sadness, confusion, or a sense of betrayal about what they are about to share. During the pause the client may request that the psychotherapist not think badly of the parent who communicated the worth-denying messaging in that particular part of the story. The client might also be compelled to pause before sharing a worth-denying memory because they are gripped by fear that they do not have permission from the parent to tell the details to someone else. In both cases, the psychotherapist is encouraged to trust the feelings that the client is experiencing in the present moment about a memorized interaction. Moreover, the client's hurt feelings need to be addressed as real before the psychotherapist can offer the client the safety of a confidential process and, if appropriate, the promise to not unfairly judge the parent from the recollection shared in session. One helpful response to a client who is afraid of hurting their parent (or the memory of the parent) by sharing their history is to ask them what part they feel comfortable to share and/or if there is something that is easier to share that will help the psychotherapist understand the memory without moving against their own values. The client may value protecting the family history, or they may believe it is disrespectful to villainize their parent when they also have positive memories of them. Consequently, the client may choose to refrain from speaking about the injunctions, especially the abusive type, if it makes the parent look bad to someone else. If the client does not feel protective or fearful about sharing their past, the psychotherapist can proceed with open-ended questions and note the naming of any injunctions that resonate with the client.

The psychotherapist who utilizes WCT constructs as a guide for exploring injunctions will first determine the client's *awareness* of the injunctions they have endured that may continue to influence their behavior. It is important to assess if the client's awareness of the injunctions they experienced in their family and/or other systems includes debilitating fear or shame. In the absence of a severe level of trauma-based fear or shame, the psychotherapist can take the time the client needs to explore their memories. In neuroscience-informed psychotherapy, emotional attunement of the psychotherapist and client includes holding a safe space for the client's verbalizations, sensations, feelings, behaviors, and knowledge that were or were not integrated in a coherent manner in childhood. This original safe organization of autobiographical memory enhances client self-awareness and increases problem-solving ability, coping ability, and affect regulation (Cozolino, 2010). A psychotherapy process that is safe and secure can invite the client's attachment circuitry to re-engage, allowing for awareness to surface. Following this awareness assessment, the client is *respect(fully)* invited to share what they are comfortable with and are provided the option of pausing if needed or ending the sharing of the event(s) in that session. Naming the injunctions may help the client see that it was the message that was handed down, and not necessarily a purposeful worth-denying assertion. However, if the injunctions were consistently and purposely abusive and not just intrusive, the client may experience parental injunctions as weapons used against them. *Esteem* is another important WCT construct in the client's exploration of injunctions. More specifically, the WCT psychotherapist holds the client in esteem as the client manages difficult memories and associated emotions in session. The client who has been exposed to intrusive or abusive injunctions that are delivered through a double-bind message (i.e., two or more reciprocally conflicting messages such as a person communicating one thing verbally, but using nonverbal language to say something completely different) may have developed the skill of reading facial expressions or listening for a change in tone of voice to discern the hidden intent of incongruent messages. Holding the client in esteem acknowledges the client's effort to find the truth and can help them recognize that they are not bad or wrong to see through conflicting communication. Lastly, the psychotherapist can assist the client in their retelling of childhood challenges by having *confidence* in the client finding their way through the old rhetoric that has caused harm and a lost-worth story. This confidence extends to the client's recognition of what is true for them, and the ability to connect that felt experience with their BSW.

The Four Pillars of Self-Worth

Learning how to build one's life in a way that consistently affirms BSW starts within the family system. Not all family systems promote unconditional affirmation of each member's BSW. Building blocks which are made of affirming moments (e.g., providing an affirming response to the child's signals) are necessary to create the four pillars of self-worth. More specifically, a worth-affirming building block is the basic unit in a pillar of self-worth. In WCT, moments of time include internal experiences which signal and receive self-worth needs and external interactions with others (first caregivers, then anyone) when a building block (a unit of affirmation) is given in response to each self-worth need.

Limitations that restrict access to building blocks for one or more members in the system can exist. Limits include caregivers not having self-worth needs met consistently or not having enough worth-affirming building blocks to construct pillars that affirm individual self-worth (this can be from a scarcity of blocks in the system). Consider the following examples, which illuminate unmet self-worth needs and the absence of worth-affirming building blocks in a family system. A family living in poverty with parents working two or three jobs each in order to make ends meet may be too tired at the end of the day to attend to the needs of their children. Sadly, these parents are barely able to provide food and shelter, let alone address self-worth needs with worth-affirming building blocks. Similarly, a parent who has not had their BSW affirmed consistently, and who conformed to the condition placed on them in childhood to be smart, is unable to support the BSW of their child who has attention deficit hyperactivity disorder because they are failing a class. In this example, the parent is stuck in the condition that gave them importance (i.e., being smart) and unable to share worth-affirming building blocks that they themselves do not have. Of further import and consistent with a two-parent household, one parent might be better at acknowledging and responding to their child's self-worth needs than the other parent. Also, one or both parents may have some worth-affirming blocks but not enough to construct pillars that affirm their own individual self-worth or the self-worth in others. If one or both parents have enough blocks to give, it could be that at the end of the day, they are successful at meeting life needs but that they lack the energy required to address additional needs (i.e., self-worth needs). A final example of restricted access to building blocks in a family is when the use of building blocks has fallen out of practice because a divorce disrupted the co-construction of worth-affirming building blocks (i.e., the parent who co-constructed using worth-affirming blocks with them is no longer accessible).

The pillars of self-worth in WCT are not static structures like a Greek temple; rather they are rebuildable (i.e. blocks can be assembled, reassembled, and repaired). We use an image depicting pillars similar to a smaller temple like the one at the Acropolis in Athens built for Nike with four classical columns (see Figure 6.1). The four pillars of self-worth are solid, but dynamic formations that family members build and rebuild in relation to others and self, over a lifetime, to honor BSW and to gain RSW throughout the process.

When a self-worth pillar is being co-constructed in childhood, a client learns which blocks affirm self-worth in distinctive ways, (i.e., awareness

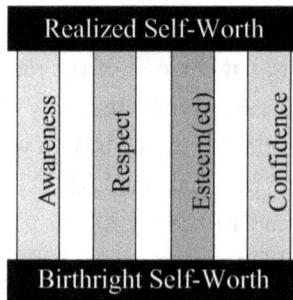

Figure 6.1 Pillars of Self-Worth.

of BSW, respect for BSW, esteem in BSW, and confidence in BSW). The client can become familiar with how to focus on BSW and later pull the best building blocks forward to be repurposed in new situations with new people. With enough worth-affirming co-construction experiences in childhood, the client can effectively employ their worth-affirming blocks in familiar and unfamiliar situations. With enough practice, recognizing and utilizing worth-affirming blocks can eventually happen effortlessly for a client; the practice becomes a pattern of behavior through building pillars of self-worth by consistently accessing the blocks that affirm self-worth which were available in the family and community systems, or which are shared in psychotherapy.

Building each pillar of self-worth corresponds with a stage of development. The stages of development described by Erikson (1950) pair up with the initial building of the pillars of self-worth through childhood. Each of Erikson's stages lays the foundation for understanding how human development occurs in sequential stages. The application of Erikson's stages is advantageous for specifying how and when the pillars of self-worth can be built when available resources for building the pillars are present in the system. Although co-construction of the pillars continues throughout the child's life, families are not always building pillars of self-worth; rather, pillars can be built on conditions instead of on BSW. A repertoire of co-construction is developed in relationships within the family system, but significant relationships outside the home can be another source for learning the necessary building skills.

Each pillar of self-worth begins with blocks that belonged to caregivers. The blocks represent moments of interaction between caregiver and child, and between the child's internal reality and the external world. Each interaction can provide a model and promote self-awareness, self-respect, self-esteem, or self-confidence. WCT proposes that awareness of BSW is essential before the individual can recognize they have something to respect. Respect as the second pillar allows a person to protect their BSW. Protecting one's BSW opens up the opportunity to experience it more regularly and to esteem what feeling worthy is like. These three pillars of self-worth bestow confidence in BSW, which can be protected with respect, and enjoyed as a basic truth.

Erikson's Developmental Stages and WCT

Erikson's theory of psychosocial development describes 8 stages, each of which represents a critical period of development in which individuals face challenges that shape their psychosocial well-being. Erikson was specifically interested in how relationships and social interactions inform the development and growth of human beings. In Table 6.2 we align the outcomes of WCT with Erikson's stages of development.

Imitation Pillars, Conditions, and Counterfeits

Although members in family systems are always using building blocks, it is important to clarify that they are not always building with blocks that promote pillars of self-worth on a foundation of BSW. Pillars built on conditions of self-worth can be built in any system that fosters the importance of a condition over the value of affirming individual BSW. A condition is a substitute for BSW that is not only allowed, but it can also be celebrated. Family members can share building blocks that affirm the condition in daily interactions, such as during a talk between a caregiver and a child. For example, a child who expresses dislike of continuing to pursue Taekwondo lessons after they have reached the competition level, may receive the following adamant response from their parent: "We are not quitters in this family!" The parent does not realize that their expectation of their child not quitting may be a condition that is replacing affirming BSW in their child. A BSW-affirming response might be "Tell me more about why you do not want to continue Taekwondo?" The parent may have experienced a positive outcome from using this value in their own life, but they are applying it to their child's situation without knowing why the child wishes to quit. The child cried after being told they could not stop participating in the competitions. The parent was not without sympathy and asked, "Why are you crying? You have loved learning Taekwondo?" The child was familiar with the idea that in this family some questions were really statements (reinforcing a condition). But the child persisted and at that point told the rest of their story, their eyes filled with tears again and they told the truth—I hate hitting people. The child further shared that it felt wrong when the coach encouraged them to hit another child during the competitions. The child did not want to

Table 6.2 Erikson's Psychosocial Stages and WCT Outcomes

Erikson's Psychosocial Stages

Stages 1–8	Conflict	Important Events	Erikson and WCT Outcomes
Infancy (Birth–18 months)	Trust vs Mistrust Trusting leads to Hope	Feeding	Trust develops through consistent care of the child. In WCT, the child begins to trust that their signals are important, and they gain self-awareness which includes awareness of feeling worthy. The consistent care by others begins the foundation of self-respect.
Early Childhood (2–3 years)	Autonomy vs Shame/Doubt Autonomy leads to Will.	Toilet Training	Self-direction develops through gaining a sense of control over physical skills. In WCT, a child grows in self-awareness and self-respect as they continue to trust giving and receiving signals. They can also start to feel esteem from others for recognizing their own signals in a timely manner.
Preschool (3–5 years)	Initiative vs Guilt Initiative leads to Purpose	Exploration	Personal power develops and is managed with feedback from others. Interests are encouraged. In WCT, the child continues to develop self-awareness, self-respect, and self-esteem. They can bring these capabilities to new interests. As they feel worthy of using the building blocks, they bring that sense of worth to things they are interested in.
School Age (6–11 years)	Industry vs Inferiority Industry leads to Competence	Education	Success in school leads to a sense of competency. In WCT, the child can experience self-confidence and begin building this final pillar of self-worth as they feel capable of learning. They can also start to demonstrate confidence in using the building blocks to build all four pillars of self-worth.

(Continued)

Table 6.2 (Continued)

Erikson's Psychosocial Stages

Stages 1–8	Conflict	Important Events	Erikson and WCT Outcomes
Adolescence (12–18 years)	Identity vs Role Confusion Identity leads to Fidelity	Social Relationships	The child gains a personal identity. In WCT, the adolescent is using building blocks from their family and adding building blocks they recognize as useful in constructing solid pillars of self-worth. They can feel true to themselves and use that awareness to act in self-respect.
Young Adult (19–40 years)	Intimacy vs Isolation Intimacy leads to Love	Relationships	The young adult knows themself well enough to share who they are without feeling compromised. In WCT, the young adult has built the four pillars of self-worth and can recognize friends and potential partners who have a solid sense of worth. They want people in their lives who will help them maintain their sense of worth. They can offer and receive worth-affirming awareness, mutual respect, appropriate praise, and confidence.
Middle Adult (40–65 years)	Generativity vs Stagnation Generativity leads to Caring	Work and Parenthood	Success leads to feelings of accomplishment in adulthood. In WCT, the adult who is able to maintain their four pillars of self-worth can share their knowledge. They will feel useful and helpful when they offer building blocks to others. Sharing their expertise on how they developed a realization of their worthiness is natural and effortless.
Mature Adult (65–Adult)	Ego Identity vs Despair Integrity leads to Wisdom	Reflection on Life	Personal fulfillment is the result of accomplishments. In WCT, enjoying the wisdom of knowing how to be true to oneself, honoring BSW in self and others, and gaining realized self-worth through maintaining the four pillars of self-worth is fulfilling. This individual has a deep and solid identity.

be a quitter (disappointing a parent), but they also did not want to be a hitter (disappointing themself).

If the child was required to persist to accept the condition (acquiring the parent's value of not quitting) they would have been moving against an inherent value (non-aggression) without understanding that this swap of gaining the parent's approval instead of honoring something true within self adds more building blocks to an imitation pillar. The imitation pillar does not support RSW; instead, it supports a counterfeit such as the approval of becoming a skilled Taekwondo athlete. The child's imitation pillar of awareness was not grounded in BSW; rather, it was built on the condition that "We don't quit," an unshared value in the moment that may become an unwelcome acquired value for the child. The child's self-respect pillar was built on the same condition because the child's inherent value (i.e., non-aggression) was not seen as a good alternative. This action of devaluing an inherent value over the parent's preferred value adds blocks to the imitation self-respect pillar, and over time, the child learns to respect their elders, respect not quitting, and respect persevering (all good things) but at the expense of what they actually value inherently. The parent is transferring their values (through sharing building blocks) without checking in with the child about how helpful the conditions are to their authentic sense of self and BSW.

Conditions of self-worth and the counterfeit they support go hand in hand (see Figure 6.2). The Taekwondo example showed that the condition for approval was that the child not quit. That behavior requirement is not a bad or unhelpful request in and of itself. However, if a parent uses intrusive or abusive injunctions to cajole or force the pursuit of the preferred goal, the adherence to the conditions in the system exacts a higher cost on worth. The requirements in the system can become more problematic, such as when the child must lose their sense of self or BSW because the price to belong thwarts realizing their worth. The counterfeit (desired goal) makes surrendering to the conditions in the system less miserable because everyone reinforces that *not quitting* is who we are as a family. The addition of injunctions (i.e., direct parental statements and attributions about 'what the child is') and competing values makes the process of enduring the conditions more miserable. Whereas quitting was unacceptable in the family system example above, quitting might

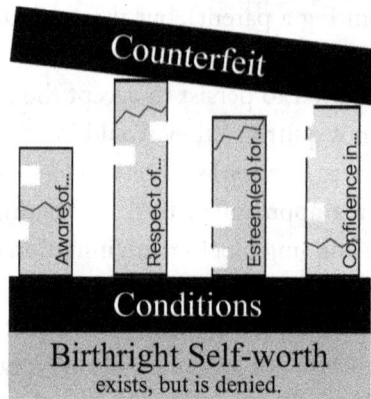

Figure 6.2 Imitation Pillars.

Note: Imitation pillars built in the service of a counterfeit are made of conditional building blocks that are prone to pillar instability due to cracks from failing conditions and BSW-affirming blocks that are missing. Imitation pillars are faulty and never solid enough for one to feel complete.

actually be an acceptable counterfeit in another system. More specifically, quitting can occur in families who have given up on trying; they may say, we cannot win. A family system may have adopted a condition such as, *People like us cannot beat the system.* The statements that might be heard in this family between members are 'You do not have to try so hard?', or 'What are you trying to prove?', or 'Stop showing off'. The members who buy into the counterfeit that the system cannot be overcome will gain awareness of how they are disempowered through the sharing of building blocks that are set up on the condition of surrender. In this system, quitting is acceptable because it supports the counterfeit (i.e., we cannot beat the system).

A WCT psychotherapist who perceives that a client is struggling to love the pillars that they have spent their life building, would not point out this struggle because it would be akin to telling the client that they have wasted years living the only way they knew how rather than building pillars that promote their BSW. Instead, the WCT psychotherapist would let the client come to that realization and then provide validation of the client's awareness. It can be challenging for some clients to fathom that what they have built does not affirm their self-worth; this can cause them to feel foolish or even overwhelmed by the realization. It is like finding out that all of your hard work was wasted. Looking at the pillars that have been built starts with identifying which of the four pillars have blocks in them that serve to prop up a counterfeit using unhelpful injunctions, acquired values, and any worth-denying beliefs that kept the client acceptable in the system.

The restrictions (i.e., conditions, injunctions, competing values, anything that keeps the client from affirming their BSW) a client rehearses in their mind will point the psychotherapist toward the counterfeit (i.e., required goal) that was held as important enough to endure the restrictions. When the counterfeit is regarded as valuable, slowly sacrificing one's sense of self becomes acceptable because something better is believed to be forthcoming. However, after successfully attaining the counterfeit, the client does not feel more worthy. The client is doing what they know how to do as well as they can, and yet they do not feel better. A simple way to look at this is that some people learn to pursue happiness by being successful at something and when they succeed the happiness gained is fleeting. Consequently, they have to always do more to feel better, but that does not translate to feeling worthy. When worthiness is seen as unnecessary or unattainable in a system, the pursuit of it may be judged pointless or foolish.

The client can take a role in the family system that is predefined and predictable giving them fictitious strength (e.g., praise or acceptability for conforming) when they have performed their role successfully, and false constraints (e.g., criticism or rejection for having self-worth needs) when they have performed their role poorly (Ferrucci, 2006). When a client has built imitation pillars on a foundation of conditions, they may live for decades before realizing that there were constraints in the system where they were raised. The lack of worth-affirming blocks available to build pillars that would have honored their BSW may remain a mystery to them because what was normalized in their family was and still is standard practice. They may start to consider that conditional building blocks inadvertently restricted the use of worth-affirming blocks, which were less available in the system. They may also recognize that BSW-affirming building blocks were not identified as valuable because they did not reinforce the preferred and well-known condition(s). The client most likely used what was abundant in the system and built what they could build. The client may look back at their childhood and piece together that they developed a habit of choosing blocks that would not burden the fragile fiction of trusting a foundation of conditions. The client can become conscious of the behaviors that served the desirable counterfeit but obscured their self-worth. The WCT psychotherapist would help the client understand that having enough BSW blocks could break through the false foundation and shock the system into an awareness of a false bottom (conditions of worth), and that not wanting to shock the system when they were younger may have been an act of kindness.

Instead of a child refraining from bringing up worth-affirming options (out of kindness) after a parent has reacted negatively to that suggestion, the child might choose to rebel. Rebellion against the conditions and refusal to participate in pursuing the counterfeit can be labeled by the parent as bad behavior or wrong choices. This type of rebellion is actually an attempt by some children to live their truth, which requires that they move against the system in order to be seen. When the child is called bad because the system supports the desired counterfeit, the child may believe they are wholly bad or wrong. Members who are compliant with the systemic requirements may use the term rebellion in a judgmental way rather than embrace it as an action against injustice for the person who resides in a non-BSW-affirming system.

It is important to note that two things can occur which encourage complicity in a system that builds and reinforces imitation pillars: (a) a child will not want to rock the boat a second time after being compelled to be more considerate of the systemic restraints (i.e., referred to as kindness); and (b) a child who rocks the boat (i.e., rebels) because they do not want to continue to be constrained by the protocol on the boat that everyone endures is called inconsiderate (i.e., criticized as the problem) by the people who do not see any problem with the protocol or the destination.

The client may have a childhood story about gaining awareness of their BSW at school, from a coach, or in a club that they excitedly shared at home with a parent, only to discover that new or different thinking that does not support the counterfeit was not considered acceptable;

consequently, the client's sharing of self-worth-based information stopped. The fictitious strengths (i.e., skills and adeptness at building impressive imitation pillars on conditions that look good and even feel good sometimes, but do not affirm self-worth) that the client gained and trusted, which allowed the conditions to prevail into adulthood, may have caused feelings of complicity that were confusing enough to seek help. Clients can feel ashamed as they grapple with the idea that their lifelong construction of pillars does not honor their whole truth or individual worth. The personal cost of denied BSW was not understood in childhood because everyone was focused on achieving the goal without knowing the price of participation. As an adult, the client, having more exposure to worth-affirming behavior in different relationships, can realize the degree of their lost sense of self. They can begin recounting the behavior that satisfied the systemic requirements, which allowed the constant disregarding of their self-worth needs.

The whole family system may have believed that once the counterfeit was reached something of worth would be obtained, but all the while, their real worth was available and waiting to be remembered. This realization can be both liberating and humiliating for some clients. It is liberating because the client knows that they have been stuck in a pattern of building pillars that has not made them feel good about themselves and has caused them to feel more self-conscious and less worth-conscious. Their newfound realization allows them to learn what is not working and what can work better to promote their wellness. On the contrary, it is humiliating to learn that the pillars they have spent a lifetime building, and which are approved in their family system and possibly also their community, do not help them to realize something about themselves that they have always possessed and that could have provided solid strength based in BSW. The psychotherapist has the complicated task of helping to liberate the client from their history and the repetition of building imitation pillars without destroying what they have built. The WCT psychotherapist will help the client repurpose building blocks that have supported imitation pillars, identify and name any blocks that can serve RSW, and co-create a new worth-conscious wellness practice with the client.

References

Berne, E. (1964). *Games people play: The basic handbook of transactional analysis*. New York: Grove Press. ISBN 0-14-002768-8.

Budiša, D., Gavrilov-Jerković, V., Dickov, A., Vučković, N., Mitrovic, S. M. (2012). The presence of injunctions in clinical and non-clinical populations. *International Journal of Transactional Analysis Research*, 3(2), 28–36 https://doi.org/10.29044/v3i2p28

Cozolino, L. (2010). *The neuroscience of psychotherapy: Healing the social brain*. New York, NY: Norton.

Erikson, E. (1950). *Childhood and society*. New York: W. W. Norton.

Ferrucci, P. (2006). *The power of kindness: The unexpected benefits of leading a compassionate life*. New York: Penguin Books/Penguin Group (USA).

Goulding, R. L., & Mary, M. (1978). *The power is in the patient*. San Francisco: TA Press.

7

THE FOUR QUADRANTS

WCT Four Quadrants

The four quadrants of WCT represent two variables coming together to show how they might shape the experience of the individuals living in systems where those variables exist to a lesser or greater extent (see Figure 7.1). The two variables are life needs, which include the two

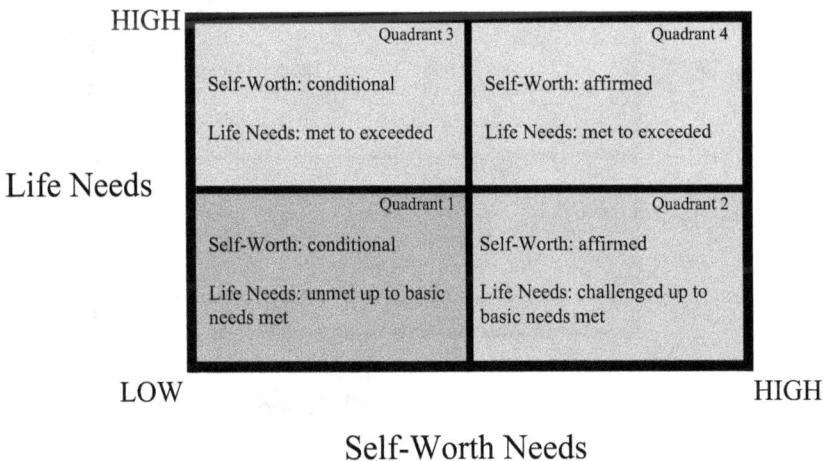

Figure 7.1 The Four Quadrants of WCT.

DOI: 10.4324/9781003599739-7

foundational levels of Maslow's hierarchy of needs (i.e., physiological and safety) and self-worth needs (i.e., awareness, respect, esteem(ed), confidence). The needs represented in Figure 7.1 can be congruent such as when both life needs and self-worth needs are met, or incongruent such as when one set of needs is met, and the other is not. Life needs and self-worth needs are also considered high or low as indicated by the extent to which they are met.

Quadrant 1 (Q1): Life needs are not met or barely being met. The lack of unmet life needs coinciding with unmet self-worth needs is descriptive of a combination of difficulties which can demoralize an individual. The struggle to have basic life needs met while being abused or ill used by others in the system sets these individuals up to believe they have no birthright, nothing of value (see Figure 7.2). Too low or the absence of life and self-worth needs make living a life in Q1 undesirable. In this quadrant, many people have been excised from family and forgotten by society such as the drug addicts living in Vancouver, Canada who were chronicled by Gabor Maté (2020). The addicts who Maté worked with seemed to be thrown away by society. Their obsessive pursuit of the next substance was seen as weakness and foolishness

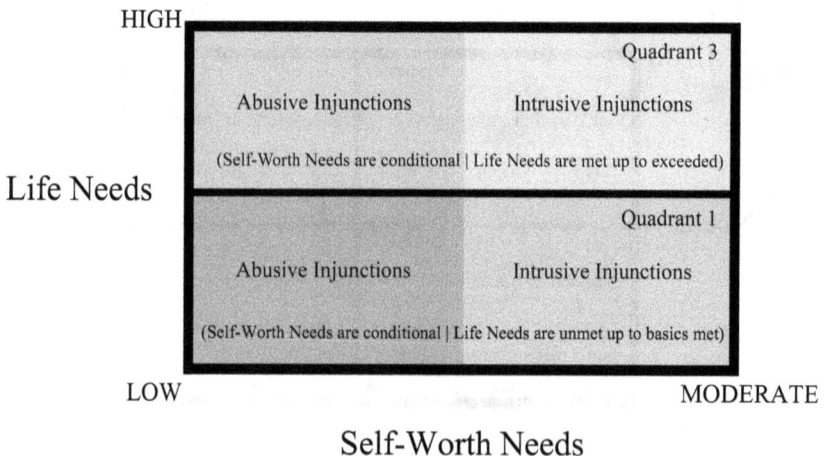

Figure 7.2 WCT Quadrants 1 and 3.

by many members of their local scene. Maté found himself face to face with patients who had a lost-worth story (LWS) that allowed them to jeopardize their next breath. We hypothesized that a commonly labeled human weakness, like believing oneself to be void of birthright self-worth (BSW) because it was denied repeatedly by family and larger systems, is frightening in its power to perpetuate a stereotype that some people are good enough or favored and others never will be. A social condition that has denied the BSW of whole groups of people is that favoritism of one person or group over another is fine, but it is actually a type of abuse. To be favored in a family or larger system a person may subjugate themselves to the leader who sets the conditions for gaining positional power in that system. The favored member's values may slip away in order to accept the required conditions, no matter if those *right conditions* infringe on the truth and worth of the member. Favored members of society who have gained some status in their families or communities may prefer to avoid noticing how fragile our humanity is toward people who did not or would not conform to the systemic conditions, and therefore did not have their basic needs and self-worth needs met. It may be easier to label those who did not conform as the problem and not the sickness in the system. The people living life in Q1 become a convenient warning to other members of the larger system. That is, members at the top of the system who wield the promise of power create the fiction that complicity to systemic favoritism is a way to be special in a system that subsequently delivers importance but denies BSW.

A benefit of living in Q3, where life needs are always met and self-worth is conditional, is that whole groups of people could be insulated from a personal or social fall from grace by means of keeping up the façade. An example of the cover-up/façade might be a fraternity that vouches for a brother to keep him from being kicked out of school by saying he was at the house the whole night. This safety from a loss of status is upheld when the exigencies (i.e., conditions, requirements, acquired values) in the system reward individual conformity (i.e., status replaces self-worth). The exchange of status (or favoritism) for worthiness is slow and unnoticeable by most children until the contract between giver and receiver is internalized (i.e., the moment when the receiver accepts the outside control and is complicit in the control over them). The poverty of unmet life needs, and self-worth needs found in Q1 reflects a place apart from grace that is full of non-conformists who eventually surrendered to the belief that what had been denied (i.e., BSW) may not have really existed.

Quadrant 2 (Q2): Although the self-worth needs of family members are met consistently, their life needs are met inconsistently or with the help of others. Because of the family system's belief in BSW, the adults in this quadrant will ask for help from larger systems to obtain food, clothing, and shelter for their family. The children are aware of the challenges the adults face (e.g., financial struggles, food insecurity, inadequate housing), but the BSW of members is promoted even when life needs are difficult to secure. The family members will talk about better days ahead, or the parent(s) may sacrifice to give their children a better life by taking additional work that pays for the higher education of the next generation. These families are aware of their BSW, respect it, have esteem for one another, and persist in the confidence that their worth will be honored if they persevere.

The leader(s) in the family systems in Q2 are aware of the difference between their children surrendering to a life outside social grace versus accepting that they are worthy of having their needs met. By endowing their children with BSW in an unwavering recognition of human dignity, they set in place a practice of affirming BSW. Investing in the BSW of the children is not conditional and status or favoritism is not used to segregate family members into categories of right or wrong based on adherence to rigid requirements that promise positional power. An example of life in Q2 includes Wanda, a mother who left an abusive partner who was the sole provider of life needs but who moved against the BSW of family members. Wanda found a home she could afford by working two jobs and she secured help through the school system to make sure her children had the meals they needed and the educational support to finish homework assignments she could not help them with. She would remind her children that they deserve a better life where they are always loved and respected.

Quadrant 3 (Q3): Life needs are met or exceeded; however, self-worth needs remain unmet by degree of severity. Exposure to abusive injunctions is more severe than having one's self-worth needs marginalized by intrusive injunctions. In this quadrant and similar to the propositions of Lamont (2019), we understand that there is a section of the population who are middle- to upper-class who may be, at worst, characterized by a frenzied pursuit of consumption and status. This pursuit for status accompanies the unchecked desire for material success that creates a contingent type of worthiness (a *having* type) that may set people up to mistakenly deny BSW (a *being* type). In WCT, we do not acknowledge the having type as a type of worthiness; it is a way to deny BSW (mistakenly or purposefully) and is a type of importance that is not worth based. The use of injunctions ranges from abusing individuals physically, sexually, emotionally, or mentally with total disregard for their BSW to intrusions that infringe on one or more family member's sense of self. Both types of injunctions (i.e., abusive and intrusive) require the use of sanctioned values (i.e., acceptable but conditional values in the system) over the discovery, development, and inclusion of an individual's inherent (i.e., individually experienced) values and also acquired (i.e., individually chosen) values that have been vetted and deemed helpful. The struggle in Q3 is that a family member may not be important in their family or community system if they rebel against the dominant conditions; in doing so, they may not recover their BSW. More specifically, a family member who rebels could move against the system and not find their inherent worth in the process; consequently, they could fall from grace, be shunned, and continue to feel unworthy. Their unmet self-worth needs may have been the reason they rebelled, but the rebellion did not secure getting those needs met. If they fall into a group of the socially disenfranchised, they may find like-mindedness in sharing lost-worth stories, but this camaraderie will not secure their BSW.

An example of someone in Q3 is Margot, a teenager from an affluent family in Arizona. Her family was adamant that there was only one way to heaven and if she did not attend church services she was physically carried to her room and left there without meals until she asked for forgiveness. This went on until Margot ran away to live with a cousin; she was only allowed to stay at her cousin's home until her mother convinced them that there was no truth to what Margot had told them and that Margot was exaggerating things. Back at her parents' house, Margot found some kids in the neighborhood who gave her alcohol and blunts when they would hang out together. She discovered that she felt less fear and anger when she used substances and that felt better than the shame her parents heaped on her whenever she resisted the conditions they loved. She had become aware of their love, respect, and esteem for heaven but not for her.

Quadrant 4 (Q4): Life needs are met or exceeded, and self-worth needs are met. Congruency between having both life and self-worth needs met creates a benefit that people living in this quadrant enjoy. They feel secure in their humanity and, because they are not facing challenges to either set of needs, they have time and energy to realize a worth-affirming existence. If a person is not born into a family or community system in this quadrant, they can migrate to it.

Migrating to Q4

A person migrating to Q4 will need to have built the majority of each pillar with worth-affirming blocks. This does not mean the person can achieve a perfect state of error-free worth-affirming behavior. The client may still include information about themselves or others that is not helpful in realizing their self-worth. They can also exclude information that is valuable to realized self-worth (RSW) or retell old stories that deny the helpfulness of self-worth as a wellness practice. When a client has built pillars of self-worth that were mostly solid, they may become more aware of mistakes and have the self-respect to acknowledge them. They can also stay open to the fact that they dislike making mistakes without losing the ability to like themselves, and also have the confidence to correct the mistake quickly or ask for help.

An example of someone migrating to Q4 is the case of Lance, who was raised by a single mother who was an addict. When Lance was sent to live with his father, his stay was cut short. His father could not handle the responsibility of having someone in his care. Lance was taken to the bus station by his neglectful father with just enough money to only make it part-way back. When he was unable to get back on the bus, Lance used some of his money to call his mother's house. He discovered that he was not a priority to either her or her partner who was living and doing drugs with her. None of the adults in his life were affirming his self-worth and his life needs were either met inconsistently, or not met at all. He found himself homeless as a teenager. He had always felt like a liability and now he was on his own. He lived homeless for a few years, doing whatever he could do to get enough money to have his next meal. Lance eventually found his way back into housed society. He pursued an education and secured employment. He liked reading and he found that he loved the philosophy of Marcus Aurelius, a Stoic philosopher and Roman emperor. One particular concept which resonated and was also reinforced by the psychotherapy he sought as an adult through a program his employer provided was that people deserved better than what he had experienced, including the lack of acknowledged BSW from both parents and the inconsistent and often-absent recognition of his basic life needs. He wanted a better life script than the one written for him as one whose worth as a person could be conveniently disregarded for a time in both his family and community system.

Lance was on a difficult journey from the beginning because he was born into a system that did not affirm BSW. He was turning his rough road into a hero's journey, a concept popularized by Joseph Campbell (1990), in which a person finds themselves in a challenging situation, experiences a revelation, and then has a transformation that brings them back to themselves with knowledge that is beneficial. Campbell, a professor of literature and monomyth theory writer, encouraged a healthier humanity by noting that the privilege of a lifetime is being who you are (Osborn, 1995). This idea pointed to being true to self no matter the hardships a person faces. Being true to self is an integral part of WCT. When we look at Lance and his story, we do not deem the challenges his parents and society allowed him to face during childhood to be appropriate to evoke his eventual well-being. Nonetheless, his motivation to affirm that he had worth that was constantly denied by others, but still present within him, speaks to the birthright nature of self-worth. As his journey to Q4 continues, he can live his truth and affirm his self-worth consistently to build a life on a solid foundation that his birthright is real and beneficial.

To review, when a client, like Lance, only knows how to build with blocks that either deny their worth or affirm their worth conditionally, they construct imitation pillars, which obscures RSW. The work that a client puts into the conditional-based pillars may leave them tired of living a life that does not feel worthy. The conditions they built pillars on were created for them by people who did not acknowledge their BSW. Instead of enjoying steady and solid pillars that reflected his truth and worth, Lance continued to prop up a counterfeit that was heavy, cumbersome, and eventually unimpressive in comparison to what was truly desired, which was realizing his own self-worth. He eventually put his life needs in his own hands and pulled any useful building blocks away from the faulty structures and from many other helpful resources, including renowned authors and philosophers, in order to build a better life for himself.

All clients moving from a quadrant where self-worth is conditional toward Q4 are on their own heroic journey to a version of self that allows their truth and worth to work together. Consider the story of a middle-aged woman, who we will call Millie, who sought counseling because she just had experienced her third breakup in a decade, and she wondered why she kept "falling for jerks." She recognized a self-destructive pattern of falling for partners who deceived her. She wanted help with setting boundaries (self-respect pillar), so she would not fall for the same type of partner again. To help her do that, the psychotherapist helped her map her level of awareness—together they looked at which blocks were already being used in her self-awareness pillar that affirmed her BSW. Millie agreed that adding the necessary self-respect blocks in psychotherapy would make sense to her because they could be linked to her increased self-awareness. The psychotherapist would look for what level of knowledge Millie had about herself and what amount of information she used that was habitually but not purposefully denying BSW.

Potential Questions to Pose to Millie and/or Other Clients:

1. How has a lack of *self-respect* allowed others to disrespect you?
2. What degree of *self-awareness* would be needed for you to address the problem?

3. How have you learned to allow a feeling of disliking yourself (low *self-esteem*) to be evidence against the existence of your BSW?

4. Did *self-confidence* exist or was the absence of self-confidence due to a pattern of distrusting yourself?

The psychotherapist would use the above categorical questions (i.e., pillars of self-worth) to help Millie become more conscious of where she has denied her BSW, and then together examine how challenging Millie's life has been when she has had to build and repair imitation pillars. The psychotherapist will explore where awareness of what is not working can be expanded to awareness of what can work. Carl Rogers (1961) wrote about the ability to be fully open in the present moment as being a quality of a mature life. That being open includes openness to who we are and how we are wired. Rogers refers to an open person as a client who "makes use of all the information their nervous system can thus supply, using it in awareness, but recognizing that their total organism may be, and often is, wiser than this awareness" (p. 191).

BSW and Differentiation

According to family systems theorist Murray Bowen (1978), differentiation of self reflects the extent to which one is able to distinguish personal feelings and thoughts from those of others in their significant and intimate networks. "Differentiation is a tangible interpersonal process that goes on between you and other people moment-to-moment. It is also a powerful individual process that shapes your thoughts, feelings, and behavior throughout the course of your life" (Schnarch, 2009, p. 88). Dr. Schnarch, a psychologist specializing in sex therapy within the relationship context, likes to use the phrase *holding on to yourself* to describe the active practice of being a differentiated person. He uses the phrase to refer to the ability of any person to maintain a sense of self-worth and clear goals in a system or relationship dynamic where sameness to fit in may be required or where avoidance or adversity is disruptive to sense of self.

Being allowed to differentiate allows a client to be an individual (not fused) in a rigid family system. The client can experience connection from members who do or do not honor their BSW. Regardless of how consistently BSW is affirmed, the client can realize their worth through activities, interests, and values that are more individualized through a process of differentiation. Schnarch's (2009) Four Points of Balance is an excellent model for becoming differentiated in a relationship where the stakes are high (i.e., rejection is possible). Bowen (1976) conducted research with family systems and discovered that some systems were in higher states of emotional reactivity like one chaotic conglomerate. The members of these families showed an absence of personal differentiation and individuals were stuck together as though the shared emotional context was super glue.

Bowen (1978) hoped that borrowing the term differentiation from biological science would make the concept consistent with natural sciences because cellular differentiation is a process where the cells individuate from each other. Bowen saw the value of a scientific principle being applied to the family system. When we think about cellular differentiation in the 21st century, we understand the outcome of an organ that is made up of cells doing different jobs. In other words, the cells specialize in performing unique roles that are different from other cells in the same organ—and yet all of them originated from a parent cell. In WCT, we propose that clients know how to become themselves over the course of development. This is best accomplished by being true to something within self that is uniquely individual, and that is not treated in the system as unacceptable because it differs from what another member values. WCT recognizes differentiation as the process of becoming a healthy version of self that has inherent origins which allow a person's truth to emerge.

Compassion during Migration

Psychologist Kristin Neff (2011) emphasized that "we don't have to earn the right to compassion: it is our birthright" (p. 12). In WCT, we regard worthiness as our birthright and compassion as the act of responding to our own and others' worthiness from this birthright. An act of compassion is not a stronger person lifting a weaker person; rather, it is a wiser person (with RSW) who recognizes your BSW and lovingly helps you remember that is has always existed. In WCT-focused psychotherapy, self-compassion is the act of a client loving themselves through the process of accurately assessing which pillars are stable. From there, the client would identify and remove any broken blocks and discover where to get solid blocks and how to situate them where needed in order to stabilize their pillars of self-worth.

Most people have experienced the feeling of loving and being loved. When a client wants to honor their BSW and develop RSW, love is not sufficient. The experience of love provides a great starting point for clients to liberate themselves from a rigid and limiting definition of self as being of little worth. When a client is able to share what love focused inward feels like, the psychotherapist will ask them if they can love the part of themself that feels unworthy (i.e., love themself for existing despite their BSW being denied) and also love the part of themself that is willing to learn to affirm BSW (i.e., love themself for being of worth no matter what). When love as self-compassion is focused on BSW and liberally applied, the work of rebuilding the four pillars of self-worth is lighter and less emotionally heavy. Love, as noble kind-heartedness, is the verbal and emotional expression of unconditional worth, which recognizes and reflects BSW. One of the most powerful and humanizing expressions is to show love as an absolute affirmation of worth. When clients gain familiarity with focusing their love inward, it can be used to examine and learn with lovingkindness about their painful history of conforming to rules and regulations, which allowed fears of unworthiness to surface and a LWS to be written.

In WCT, we promote the idea of psychotherapists having rational compassion. Researcher Kevin Dickinson (2022) wrote about rational compassion and further explained how empathy without understanding could bias the best of good intentions. Dickinson showed that by soliciting feedback from people in the culture before taking action, the organizations interested in developing good philanthropic plans could learn how to predict any bad design consequences and better understand the communities they intended to serve. Rational compassion allows the psychotherapist and client to work together to co-create a structure (i.e., building blocks and pillars) that can fend off the overwhelming emotional state of a client who feels unworthy. Instead of relying on emotional empathy as the only guide, the psychotherapist can check in with the client about how using different building blocks to affirm self-worth will work for them and if they can take these skills home or not.

Compassion (i.e., empathetic caring) can be balanced using reason and rational thinking through the evaluation process and continue into the planning phase of psychotherapy with the client informing the psychotherapist about the system they will return to with their new building skills. Donald Winnicott, an English psychoanalyst and pediatrician, was instructive in the processes which shape neural structures. He offered the perspective that psychotherapy for the client is a process of controlled regression into childhood with the purpose of helping the client develop a true self in the present, which was obstructed in early life (as cited in St. Clair, 1986). Rational compassion as a therapeutic process addresses what is loving and caring for the client, while not ignoring what is also useful or not to their true self.

References

Bowen, M. (1976). Theory in the practice of psychotherapy. In P. J. Guerin Jr. (Ed.), *Family therapy: Theory and practice* (pp. 42–90). New York: Gardner Press.
Bowen, M. (1978). *Family therapy in clinical practice*. New York: Jason Aronson.
Campbell, J. (1990). *The Hero's Journey*. San Francisco: Harper Collins.
Dickinson, K. (2022). Why social design projects fail. *The Learning Curve Column: Big Think*. https://bigthink.com/the-learning-curve/why-social-design-projects-fail/
Lamont, M. (2019). From 'having' to 'being': Self-worth and the current crisis of American Society. *The British Journal of Sociology*, 70(3).
Maté, G. (2020). *In the realm of hungry ghosts: Close encounters with addiction*. North Atlantic Books Ergos Institute.
Neff, K. (2011). *Self-compassion: Stop beating yourself up and leave insecurity behind*. New York: HarperCollins.
Osborn, D. K. (1995). *A Joseph Campbell companion: Reflections on the art of living (1st Harper Perennial)*. Harper Perennial.
Rogers, C. R. (1961). *On Becoming a Person: A Therapist's View of Psychotherapy*. Boston, MA: Houghton Mifflin Company.
Schnarch, D. M. (2009). *Intimacy & desire: Awaken the passion in your relationship*. New York: Beaufort Books.
St. Clair, M. (1986). *Object relations and self-psychology*. Monterey, CA: Brooks/Cole.

8

PSYCHOTHERAPY TECHNIQUES

Conscious Moment Technique and Chart

The first technique established in worth-conscious theory (WCT) is the conscious moment technique (see Figure 8.1). This technique can be used in psychotherapy sessions with clients who mention having feelings of unworthiness or beliefs that they are worthless, which allows for the existence and practice of a self-conscious frame of reference. The conscious moment technique is a modified version of the Choice Point Model used in acceptance and commitment therapy (ACT). Hayes (2004) created ACT as a treatment focused on increasing client psychological flexibility in the present moment to help change or support client actions, which serve their valued outcome. ACT places emphasis on the client's values or valued goal during treatment as a necessary component of creating meaning in life (Hayes, 2004). The Choice Point Model was originally created for use by clinicians trained in the ACT approach. Harris (2019) is a proponent of using the Choice Point Model with clients because he views the model as a practical way for clients to see a visual representation of possible moves they can choose toward what they value. Moreover, as a therapeutic tool, Choice Point "…rapidly maps out problems, identifies sources of suffering, and formulates an ACT approach to handling them" (Harris, 2019, p. 9). The Choice Point Model (Ciarrocchi et al. 2013,

DOI: 10.4324/9781003599739-8

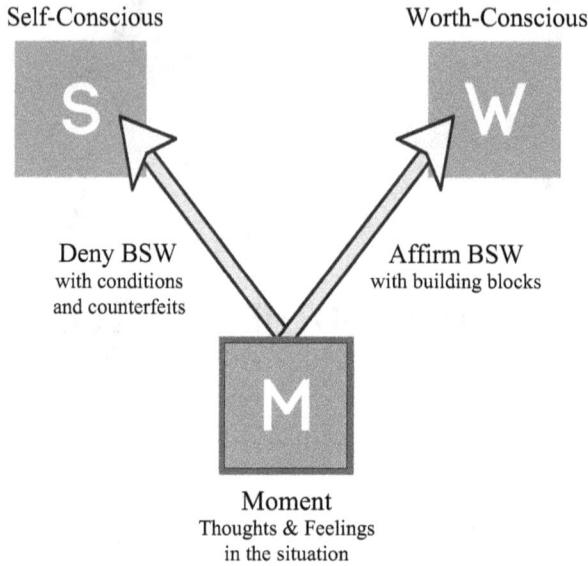

Figure 8.1 Conscious Moment Technique.

Harris, 2019; see Figure 8.2) was an excellent visual option to use as a starting point to build a WCT-based technique due to focus on the distinct point in time when a decision can be made, and consciousness can be expanded.

Conscious moment technique as a WCT modification of the Choice Point Model involves specifying that the valued outcome is birthright self-worth (BSW) and that in any given moment a client can use blocks that make up the four pillars of self-worth to affirm BSW. BSW is seen as a core value in humanity and therefore deserves recognition as something to notice, respect, esteem, and have confidence in. In WCT, the conscious moment technique is used to bring awareness to the moment when a client is retelling an unhelpful story that includes denied self-worth as more relevant than affirming BSW. Not all clients will have a lost-worth story (LWS), but when a client is repeating a personal narrative about feeling worthless, they may be reading from a worth-denying life script that is part of their stored memory, which allows for a self-conscious frame of reference. A client can become fused with any part of their history that denies their BSW. ACT seeks to undermine an attachment to a

The choice is away
from what is valued.

The choice is towards
what is valued.

Hooked

Unhooked

The
Choice
Point

A choice can be made about
the situation, thought or feeling.

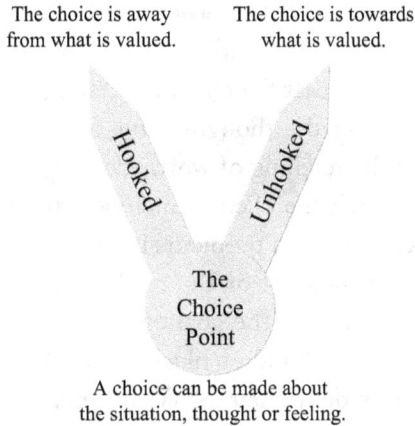

Figure 8.2 The Choice Point.

conceptualized self (i.e., a client's fused, evaluative stories about who they are) and instead promotes contact with a sense of self based on the "I/here/nowness" of conscious experience (Hayes et al., 2013, p. 7).

The WCT-trained psychotherapist using this conscious moment technique can provide the client with the option to recognize and choose thoughts, feelings, and actions that either affirm or deny self-worth by showing the client the picture of the chart as a visual tool that reinforces present moment awareness. The technique is similar to the Choice Point Model in that it includes a circle in the center bottom of the picture representing a moment when a choice can be made, with two arrows pointing upwards at opposite angles representing two distinctly different possibilities from an originating moment of consciousness. In Choice Point, the right-side arrow, designated as unhooking, is about making a choice to move in a direction that the client values and away from something that has hooked them (e.g., addiction, bad habit). The left arrow, designated as hooked, points away from those values and into what hooks the client into problematic behavior.

The WCT modification of the Choice Point Model (i.e., conscious moment technique) includes that self-worth, especially BSW, is something clients can value but which they may not have learned how to consistently affirm. In line with the Choice Point Model, the conscious moment technique also invites the client to be present, open, and to do what matters in affirming what they value, but this moment of consciousness is specific to valuing their individual self-worth. Being present in the moment might mean that the client is detailing a problem they have faced, while also sharing the thoughts and feelings they are currently experiencing during the retelling of worth-denying details. It might also be the moment at which the client remembers the thoughts and feelings they experienced during a problem situation. The client can choose to process the current moment or the remembered moment using the conscious moment technique. The goal of this technique is to assist the client with examining their building blocks in order to determine if those blocks either affirm or deny their BSW. If determined that the client has blocks that are based on the conditions in the family system, the psychotherapist can invite the client to rewrite the language or scripting associated with each block so they can turn worth-denying blocks into worth-affirming moments.

When a WCT psychotherapist uses the conscious moment technique, they can invite a client to open up in the moment to process if they are (or are not) being worth-affirming or are accidentally or habitually using worth-denying beliefs or behaviors. The client is invited to: (1) be in the moment; (2) be open to having more awareness of affirmed or denied self-worth; and (3) stay open to recognizing the options they have used that deny self-worth (such as conditions and counterfeits) or that affirm BSW. The desired openness includes: (4) considering new ways to look at decision-making; and (5) how to use thoughts, feelings, and actions they have already used (their useful building blocks) in past situations to help them affirm their BSW or any developed realized self-worth (RSW) in this moment. The psychotherapist can share better building blocks (see Figure 8.3) with the client when the client is unsure of which of their building blocks to use. Addressing which building blocks are helpful or not can begin when a client shares a situation where they have felt unworthy, and in which they did not know how to affirm their self-worth easily or without having it challenged by others at the time. The psychotherapist can invite the client to think about that same situation and how it might have been navigated by their favorite character in a show or book (or how a friend or family member handled something similar in a way

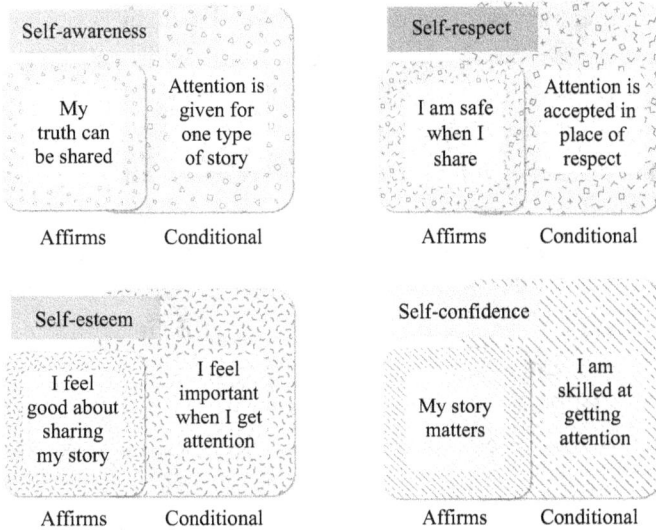

Figure 8.3 Better Building Blocks.

that the client admired). To support the client in looking for blocks they respect and are already aware of, the psychotherapist and client will assess the admired behavior (i.e., new blocks) based on worth-affirming aspects prior to the client keeping the new blocks. From there, the client will use the worth-affirming script that is amenable with the blocks they want to use and adjust the response they want to make to an option or version in which they can comfortably invest. Because building blocks are thoughts, feelings, and actions in the moment, they are informed with definitions of use, which means language can be introduced to describe the client's feelings and reactions. In other words, a client may not know why they use or have a certain set reaction, but they can use language to describe the reaction.

The confidence in using the new blocks (e.g., awareness that is more accurate, self-respect that is desired and employed, esteem that is worth-based and feels empowering, and confidence that makes the person proud in that moment) is not well-established; thus, it needs to be understood that what can be role-played in session may feel safer than what can be accomplished in a real-world setting. Together, the client and psychotherapist can also look at each of the client's previously used blocks and determine which, if any, have worth-affirming properties or potential and thus could be used to build one or more of the four pillars of self-worth. If it is determined that the client's building blocks promoted a condition instead of affirming their BSW, then an early step in psychotherapy would be to promote client awareness about how their family script for using conditional blocks was required and sustained. The next step would be to offer changes to the scripted condition-promoting language (blocks) into worth-affirming language that is familiar. Consider the following example of a client who now, as an adult, becomes aware of the conditional building blocks that were required of them during their childhood to feel special in their family system. As a child, the client received attention from a parent when they were victimized at school by the classroom bully. As the client grew up, they did not realize that they unintentionally created new bullies in new classrooms and in their neighborhood in order to continue to receive special attention (i.e., feel importance) from that parent. In this example, the condition that was built in this family system was that extra attention was given to the child for telling their underdog (i.e., victim) stories. Hence, in their pursuit for attention, the child learned to perpetuate being a victim so that they would have something interesting to share with their parent who would listen and commiserate with them. This continued for years and into adulthood until the client realized, with help from a trusted life partner, that their parent seemed unaware of the limitation imposed in conversations with them. The adult client could see that they were not given the same special attention when other life events were shared with that parent. The client, as an adult, had become tired of telling the same type of victim-oriented story and wanted to share other life events based in their truth and still be worthy of attention.

Based on the above example, the psychotherapist and client would look at the desired awareness blocks that the client hoped to use in order to establish a mutually respectful interaction with the parent that is based in their truth. The adult client has some self-awareness but not enough self-respect blocks to begin a healthier conversation. That is, they do not know how to be respected or esteemed when they share a story that the parent is not interested in hearing. They want to connect with the parent and share their life with them, but without habitually perpetuating the required condition, which is to be an underdog with a victim story in order to receive attention and feel special. Each better building block that the client wants to use in their communications with their parent can affirm the BSW of both of them. The conscious moment technique assists the client to evaluate which blocks (thoughts, feelings, words) can be helpful to affirming their BSW while also not denying their parent's BSW.

Next (6), doing what matters, is part of the conscious moment technique because it includes choosing building blocks from the four pillars of self-worth that will work to affirm BSW or RSW in any situation. The client can use their own or borrowed building blocks (i.e., those learned in psychotherapy, self-help books, character in a show or friend who handled a situation well). This awareness-growing technique allows the client to experience self-respect when they (7) practice pulling different building blocks forward and using them "as if" the problematic situation could be rewritten with actions that always affirm client self-worth. The repetition of this process can add to a sense of esteem for building worth-affirming pillars and ultimately result in the confidence to shift from scripted conditions to chosen worth consciousness.

Prior to using the conscious moment technique, the psychotherapist has discussed with the client the existence of a LWS that can subsist underneath a personal narrative. The psychotherapist will inform the client that a LWS can intrude on the personal life narrative outside of the client's awareness. Teaching the client about WCT and that a LWS can be counterproductive is a helpful preliminary psychoeducation task prior to using the technique. During a difficult decision-making moment in session, when feelings of unworthiness show up, a client who already understands (through psychoeducation) that WCT helps to repair self-worth, may feel the beginning of self-confidence in their ability to use the technique to help rewrite their LWS into a worth-affirming narrative.

Perspective Shift Technique

Clients who are experiencing discomfort, distress, and unwellness may need to shift their perspective so they can successfully embrace a new perspective that will allow both their truth and their worth to co-exist.

In WCT, we introduce the perspective shift technique which encourages psychotherapists to listen for the absence of BSW, assess for the existence of a LWS, learn how severely the LWS affects the client's quality of life, and provide BSW-affirming processes to shift the client away from a pattern of denied self-worth. For example, consider the experience of shame, which is an anti-worth experience. It is generally defined as a negative frame of reference where devaluation is accepted. Psychologists Tangney and Dearing (2002) described shame as strong negative emotions in which the feeling of global self-evisceration is experienced. The experience of shame over time may exact the highest price of total surrender to a life of denied BSW. In WCT, we say there is no good reason to stay in a state of shame. Instead, we believe a client can learn from shame-based experiences and return to understanding and affirming their BSW. When the experience of fear or shame surfaces for a client, it is essential that the psychotherapist assess for the degree of severity and for whether or not the client is also experiencing trauma. After assessing and managing the client's trauma with standardized trauma-informed techniques, the simple perspective-shifting technique can be introduced to assist the client in gaining systemic awareness and self-awareness that will make space for truth and worth to coexist.

Once a trauma-based pre-conscious schema has been co-managed and the client's nervous system is regulated (i.e., not aroused), the psychotherapist can attend to helping the client maintain an optimal state that allows for conscious thought processing so that they can proceed with introducing the perspective shift technique. Even when a trauma reaction is absent, working with a client's LWS can cause strong emotions to surface, which may cause the client to feel uncomfortable. We suggest setting up the window of tolerance or zone of optimal arousal (Siegel, 1999) as a point of reference to check in with the client as needed during the administration of the perspective shift technique. The window of tolerance is a visual aid that can be used during session to remind the client to take a break so that they can remain conscious in the work at the present moment (see Figure 8.4). The client can dictate the length of the break and the actions within the break. In addition, the psychotherapist and client can co-create the type of pause that helps the client catch their breath

Hyper-Arousal

Anxiety Anger Overwhelm High Energy
Hypervigilence Fight/Flight Chaotic

⬇

Window of Tolerance

Grounded Flexible Open/Curious Present
Able to Emotionally Self-Regulate

⬆

Hypo-Arousal

Shut Down Numb Depression
Passive Withdrawn Freeze Shame

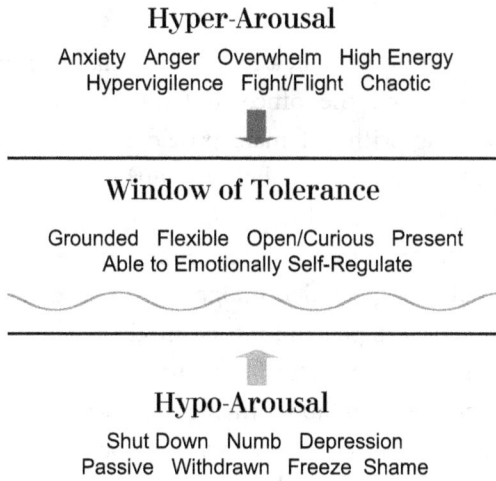

Figure 8.4 Window of Tolerance.

and return to a state of optimal arousal (i.e., alert and capable) where they feel safe enough and regulated enough to continue processing their LWS.

To help the client effectively reenter their window of tolerance, several tools may be utilized: (a) a five-count breathing exercise for two to five minutes to promote calmness; (b) a soothing technique that the client has previously found helpful; (c) standing and stretching exercises to release pent-up energy; and (d) allowing the client to express their frustrations regarding aspects of psychotherapy that trigger more anxiety, which can aid in managing their anxious energy. The psychotherapist can observe and identify when the client leaves their window of tolerance; together, they can initiate the calming or releasing activities that have helped the client to return to safe bounds before continuing the session.

Applying the Perspective Shift Technique in WCT-Focused Psychotherapy

Setting

We are at a psychotherapy group practice office that caters to a wide variety of client needs based on the specialties of counseling professionals providing client services. In addition to the utility of varied theoretical models, WCT techniques are provided as part of an overall mental health and wellness protocol.

Meeting the Client

Henrietta (they/them pronouns), a bisexual woman working as a radio-logic technologist, called the office and left a voicemail requesting immediate counseling with a female provider who understands trust and self-worth. Henrietta wanted help in getting out of a volatile relationship with their boyfriend. The psychotherapist who was assigned to work with Henrietta was a middle-aged woman named Ms. Green (she/her pronouns). Following a quick phone call to schedule the appointment, Henrietta arrived in person for their intake session. Prior to beginning the intake session, Henrietta filled out the necessary forms which included answering questions about their history and what brought them into psychotherapy at that time. They wrote about the verbal and emotional abuse they had experienced in their dating relationship and how they would freeze up whenever they heard their partner's voice start to rise in volume. They also shared the insight that they complied too easily when confronted.

Intake and Session 1

At the beginning of the session, Ms. Green walked the client through the specifics of the necessary forms, which included limits of confidentiality, billing, insurance, and a worth-conscious concept (i.e., building the self-respect pillar) was verbalized as a way to proceed to work together. Worth-conscious concepts are rooted in the building blocks from the four pillars of self-worth which can be shared by the psychotherapist throughout the psychotherapy process.

Ms. Green: May I call you Henrietta in our work together?

Henrietta: Yes.

Ms. Green: One of the rules I have for myself in our work together is to always treat you with respect. So, if anything is said in a way that changes that experience for you, please let me know and I will seek to understand what I need to do differently in order to ensure that you feel respected during our work together.

Henrietta: Nobody's ever said that to me before. I can get used to that (a positive but surprised look is on their face).

Ms. Green: Okay. One more thing, as a client you can say whatever you need to say, any way you need to say it, at the pace that makes sense for you. Is that okay with you?

Henrietta: Yes. Should I start?

Ms. Green: Yes, you can start.

During the rest of the session, Henrietta described a four-year relationship that started out as fun and easy but changed as soon as they moved in together. As partners, they have different ideas about how to spend free time and when to make time for each other. These different ideas, among others, have led to arguments with their partner, which Henrietta experiences as overwhelming. Henrietta feels different because they identify as bisexual, but their parents are only accepting of a heterosexual identity, which causes Henrietta to feel conflicted about their truth versus what their parents are accepting of and who they expect Henrietta to date. Going along with their family values felt good until recently, when Henrietta's partner yelled at them for not embracing their parents' values, which are similar to the values that Henrietta's partner espouses. Henrietta explained that the fear of being humiliated for revealing that they do not share their parents' values has become obvious whenever Henrietta starts driving home from work to meet up with their partner and have dinner with family. A sense of dread surfaces on the drive and Henrietta feels anxious about having to repeatedly explain to their partner why they feel and think the way they do. Henrietta uttered that they have not let themselves think through all of their feelings and wants help in doing that.

Psychotherapy Sessions Proceed

After a few sessions with Henrietta, Ms. Green learned that Henrietta's fear-based thinking (i.e. fear of being rejected and/or mocked for living their truth) started in childhood. As a teen, they thought both guys and girls were cute and when they were talking with friends about characters from a television show that they each liked, Henrietta shared their attraction to both a male and a female character. They did not realize that their father overheard the conversation and discussed the issue with their mother. Both parents told Henrietta that it is stupid and irresponsible to let ideas like that creep into their head. The parents continued extolling the conditions that they expected all of their children to follow. The rules they especially drilled down were about what cannot happen and what will not be tolerated. Henrietta remembered shutting down and trying to shut off their feelings.

Henrietta shared additional history in a few more sessions with Ms. Green. Throughout the sessions, they became comfortable talking about how they avoided dating during high school and got into a special program that fast-tracked students who were interested in a medical field. This was noticed and celebrated by their parents, who verbalized support and offered praise for the decision. Henrietta wanted the psychotherapist to know they loved and honored their family and that they wanted their parents to be proud of them. The need to be someone who their parents could be proud of seemed to be what led Henrietta to date someone their parents introduced them to and approved of. Henrietta finally shared that they feel stuck with a partner their parents recommended and who does not listen to, or seem to care about, Henrietta's values. Henrietta does not see a way forward that does not disappoint their parents. Ms. Green attends to the possibility that Henrietta is experiencing internal conflict between the acquired values set by their family system and their inherent values which have been pushed aside.

Initiating Perspective Shift Technique Phase 1: Listening

- The psychotherapist will begin learning about the client and listening for a LWS. This process may take three or more sessions.
- The psychotherapist will follow the pace of the client while attending with immediacy to any emergency or trauma. In the event that a client reexperiences trauma when they share aspects of a LWS, it is important that the psychotherapist follow the safety protocol they are most familiar with and trained in. For example, trauma-informed care can be used to help the client feel safe in session (see Chapter 5 for specific trauma-informed care techniques).
- The psychotherapist will use the technique of information gathering from a modality they are most comfortable with, such as motivational interviewing, cognitive behavioral therapy, dialectical

behavior therapy, acceptance and commitment therapy, narrative therapy, or another option in order to harvest aspects of the client's LWS and accompanying severity (see Chapter 5, Disrupted Well-being and Coping Chart).

- Using the information gathered, the psychotherapist becomes familiar with the client's LWS and the potential for a worth-denying mentality. In the case of Henrietta, the psychotherapist recognized that they felt trapped in a situation that stemmed from two sources. First, their partner was unkind to them but remained acceptable to the family. Second, they did not always feel acceptable in their own family. While being mindful of a few elements in Henrietta's LWS, the psychotherapist takes note of the two situations that Henrietta described as making them feel trapped as those situations may be part of a worth-denying mentality of which they are unaware, but which is common in the family system in which they grew up.
- The psychotherapist seeks confirmation that a LWS exists. As related to Henrietta, the psychotherapist sensed that they did not know how to protect themselves and their family and to stay in a close relationship with their parents. This suggested that a worth-denying mentality may exist since Henrietta feels more responsible for the approval of others than for their own BSW.

The psychotherapist listens for the degree of awareness that Henrietta has about any worth-denying messages and their own repertoire of worth-denying behaviors. Specific to Henrietta, Ms. Green recognized their emphasis on the fear-based emotion that has been attached to the verbal abuse they experienced by their partner, but that they do not seem to be attached to the worth-denying messaging in their family system.

Fifth Session—Client-Revealed Self-Worth-Denying History

After entering the psychotherapy office, Henrietta sat down and asked if they could say what was on their mind instead of picking up where they left off in the last session. Ms. Green sensed an urgency in Henrietta's face and tone of voice and agreed to the request.

Henrietta: This was on my mind the whole drive here today, so I think I need to say it out loud. I love my partner, but I am not in love with my partner. I love life, but I am not in love with my life (Henrietta started to cry). I love my family, more than I can say, but it's not enough.

Ms. Green: That sounds like a lot of strong feelings with both good and bad aspects.

Henrietta: Yeah, love is good, right (rhetorical question)? Love makes everything better, right? But it doesn't or it isn't making anything better in my life.

Ms. Green: I am hearing that there are many things you love and that you thought that would make something different or better.

Henrietta: (fear appears in their eyes) What am I doing wrong!? I must be doing something wrong! I can't get it right! (tears stream down their face and they seem frozen) My boyfriend gets so mad at me when I complain and cry and can't tell him what is wrong.

Ms. Green: Is this a place where you feel sort of stuck?

Henrietta: (cries and nods) Yeah, yeah.

Ms. Green: Are you stuck trying to do something good, like loving people, but it's not fixing what you hoped it would fix?

Henrietta: (looks up, thinks for a minute) Yeah, if my love doesn't work, what works? That's the best thing I can give. It (love) is the best thing to give, but it's not working.

Ms. Green: May I offer a summary here of what I think I am hearing you say?

Henrietta: Yeah, sure.

Ms. Green: You are trying your best to give something you believe is good (love) and that hasn't solved a problem you thought it would solve.

Henrietta: (nodding) Yeah, yeah. (face scrunched up to fight back tears) Give me a minute.

(Ms. Green pauses with Henrietta to make room and time for a strong emotion as it surfaces.)

Henrietta: (took a breath) Okay, I'm okay. We can keep going.

Ms. Green:	I have heard what you've been trying to do to solve the problem. Do I know what problem you are trying to solve?
Henrietta:	(breaks into sobs) I don't like to talk about it.
Ms. Green:	Have you talked to yourself about it before?
Henrietta:	It's been a long time. I try not to think about it.
Ms. Green:	Are you thinking about it now?
Henrietta:	Yup, it's here—full force (Henrietta appears frustrated).
Ms. Green:	Is it something you have words for today?
Henrietta:	(bursts into a statement) No matter how hard I try to be loving it's worthless. It's worthless and it is all I have to give. What is worth it then? What? What?
Ms. Green:	It sounds like you have given the best you have to give and it's not enough, and that leaves you feeling stuck in a space that allows your worthiness to be questioned.
Henrietta:	It sucks to be me!

Over the next several sessions, Henrietta shared the fear of being themself in a family that does not believe that being bisexual is possible. Their parents have said that people like that are confused, crazy, or wicked, which made Henrietta feel more unworthy. Henrietta started to recognize that when they chose pronouns in college it was fun but also a reflection of the duality they felt. That label was acceptable to some of their friends, who thought it was cool to have a choice about pronouns. Henrietta did not go into detail with all of their friends about the felt experience that made the pronoun resonate. In a later session, Henrietta shared that their boyfriend thinks it is a stupid trend (choosing pronouns) and that they should stop introducing themselves that way because it was weird, especially because they have never used them around their family.

By the seventh session, Henrietta was able to name that they felt stuck between loving their family, especially their parents, and not feeling lovable in return. The fear that they are not lovable as they are (bisexual) has affected their self-worth and kept them from telling their truth to the people who matter the most to them, which has caused an additional negative impact on their self-worth. Henrietta was able to articulate that they feel pulled to keep their parents happy, to stay in their romantic relationship, and not make people worry about them (conditions in their family system). Feeling stuck in some ways (hiding their truth in every situation) and pulled in other ways (accepting the conditions of worth in their family system) was becoming unbearable for Henrietta.

Initiating Perspective Shift Technique Phase 2: Learning

- The psychotherapist attempts to learn more about the client and what has brought them to psychotherapy. The client is invited to detail their experience and accompanying feelings. Specific to Henrietta, the psychotherapist learned that Henrietta's feelings of stuckness (i.e., hiding their truth and accepting conditions of worth) have resulted in them feeling unlovable and unworthy. The psychotherapist invited Henrietta to say more about those feelings.
- With confirmation that a story involving denied worth exists (i.e., LWS), the psychotherapist, using the information shared by the client, introduces the notion of a LWS to the client. As related to the information shared by Henrietta, Ms. Green pointed out that Henrietta's unconditional love for their family was an important and top-priority value; however, that same value was not reciprocated to Henrietta which made them feel unworthy.
- The existence of a LWS points to two poles at play. Using information shared by the client, the psychotherapist will help the client to understand how they are stuck between two poles, both of which are in opposition to their BSW. More specifically, the choice between complying with abusive injunctions against the client's truth, or accepting conditions of worth in their family system, leaves the client feeling unworthy and unable to live their truth. The psychotherapist further explains to the client that to stay stuck between two poles, neither of which support their BSW, is to accept a LWS as the only narrative available to them. In exploring the experience of feeling stuck with Henrietta, Ms. Green asked if they could explain what they were feeling. Henrietta's simple but profound statement was "it sucks to be me;" they alluded to a mental and emotional space where they have tried and failed to be worthy within their family system. Hence, Henrietta continues

to pretend, at home and in new relationships, that they are not bisexual. Henrietta keeps the pretense up because it has become well-practiced and also because pretending keeps them safe from rejection. The resulting consequence of Henrietta's experience of denied self-worth in their family system is the loss of truth and worth as a person. Finally, Henrietta reminded Ms. Green that, unlike their family members, they would not impose conditions of worth on the people they love.

- Following confirmation of the client's experience of *stuckness and when the emotions accompanied by their revelation of unworthiness have calmed, the psychotherapist can begin to attend to the client's idea of stuckness as a major component of a LWS. The psychotherapist understands that the unveiling of a LWS occurs slowly and carefully as it is quite likely that the client hates having a LWS and has probably avoided the feelings attached to it. During the session when the client feels brave enough/ready enough, they will tell themselves the truth about having their truth and worth denied. It is a good idea to check in with the client about their readiness to proceed to learn about the dynamics of their LWS before the psychotherapist maps it out with the client. Once the client is interested in learning about their LWS, the psychotherapist can use visual aids, such as the different stages of the perspective shift technique presented in Figure 8.5. Specifically, two circles can be drawn to represent the two poles in the perspective shift technique. One pole/circle symbolizes the worst worth-denying experiences in the client's life (i.e., complying with injunctions and not living one's truth), and the other pole/circle symbolizes the experiences that seem better because worth is not overtly denied, but it is conditional (i.e., living the acquired values and accepting the conditions and counterfeits required in the system).

*The learning phase of the perspective shift technique is initiated when the client feels stuck in one of the poles or between two poles. However, the psychotherapist may identify that, in the absence of the client feeling stuck, the client experiences mild to

Phase 1:
Listening

LWS

Listen for the existence
of the client's LWS.

Phase 2:
Learning

Worst — Better

Denied worth
and truth.

Conditional worth,
discounted truth.

Learn about the poles
in the client's LWS.

Phase 3:
Understanding

Worst — Me — Better

Acknowledge both
denied worth and truth.

Acknowledge
conditional worth
and discounted truth.

Summarize the LWS
and the stagnation
in one pole or
cycle between poles.

Introduce a third position.

Phase 4:
Gaining
worth-consciousnes

Overcoming
the worst — BSW — Becoming
better/best

Being

Shift away from
denying worth and truth.

Shift toward affirming
worth and truth
without conditions.

Reframe the poles as
opportunities for
worth-based growth.

Support BSW as
part of being human.

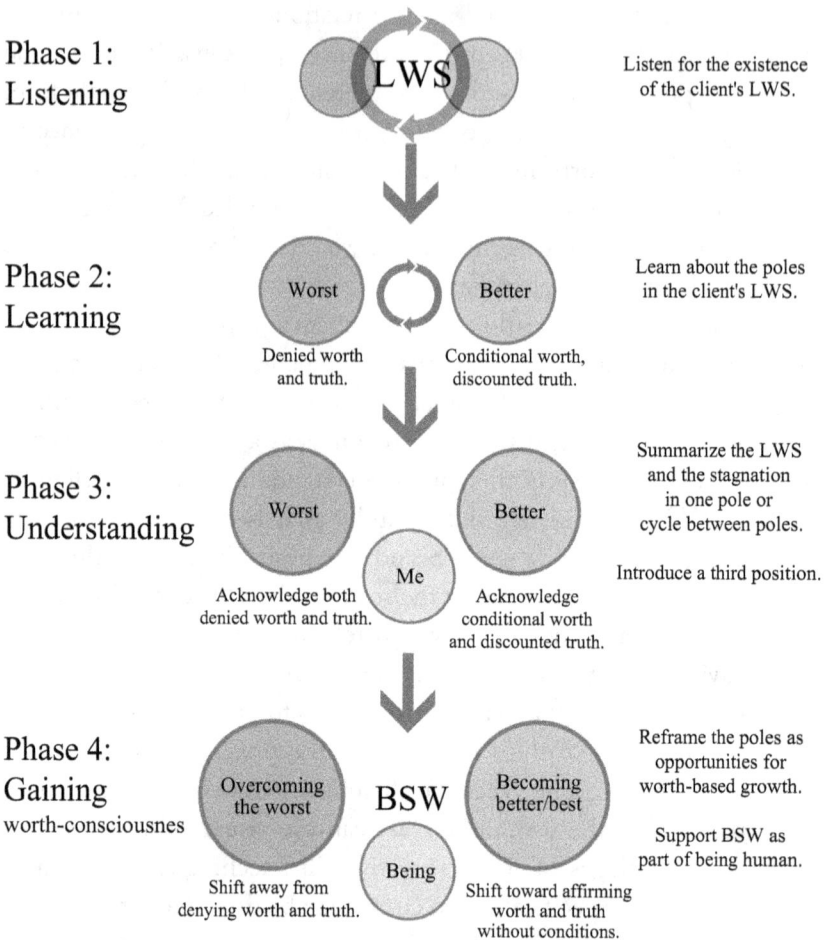

Figure 8.5 Perspective Shift Technique.

moderate conditions on their worth with a counterfeit that makes
them feel important but not worthy. In this circumstance, just one
of the poles would exist and although the client may not hate their
life, they can feel frustrated trying to succeed in a family system
that imposes conditions of worth. Thus, the client who does not
exhibit feeling stuck in one or between two poles can still benefit from the learning phase of the perspective shift technique by
focusing on the lesser degree of compliance expected in the one
pole where conditions of worth and discounted truth are imposed.

- The psychotherapist will use the details the client has provided to categorize the different worth-denying experiences into one of the two poles. Throughout sessions, the client can continue to share memories that can be placed into either category. The client may report that they feel stuck in one pole more than the other, or they may feel equally frustrated by being pushed and pulled in their family system between two poles that are both in opposition to their BSW. In working with Henrietta, Ms. Green uses a pen and paper to encourage Henrietta to write down their memories. Writing can help clients to focus and engage their thinking, which can help to capture the client's remembered experiences (Konnikova, 2014). In subsequent sessions, Henrietta is encouraged to continue to recall and map out both internal (i.e., becoming complicit and adopting the systemic requirements) and external (i.e., circumstances in the system that impact the client) events that have repeatedly denied their self-worth and inherent values in their family system. Henrietta's recall and mapping process includes identifying any pattern of denial they have experienced in their relationship with their partner. Some of Henrietta's BSW-denying events (thoughts, feelings, actions) have been committed against Henrietta by their loved ones (i.e., external). Some of the events that Henrietta experienced were repetitions of habitual compliance to requirements that Henrietta engaged in without full awareness of committing worth-denying actions (i.e., internal) against themself.

Reviewing Phases 1 and 2 and Preparing for Perspective Shift Technique Phase 3: Understanding

We have previously mentioned that some clients will have a conditional worth story that has frustrated them but not made them feel trapped. The third phase of the perspective shift technique is to understand the stuckness of a client with a LWS. Although processing a conditional worth story can also happen during this phase, it is less likely that the client's story has caused them to lose their sense of direction (i.e., feel stuck). An awareness of and respect for self-worth and lived truth provide a sense of direction. They also give rise to feelings of self-esteem and confidence, which are grounded in the congruency that these core concepts cocreate.

The psychotherapist and client have spent multiple sessions together listening to and learning about the client's LWS. At this point they have mapped out key aspects of the type of stuckness felt by the client. This can include feeling stuck in one of the poles, or between the two poles. A client can feel pulled into a pattern of conditions and counterfeits that are placed on all members of the family (a better but not healthier pole) or pushed into a pattern of abusive injunctions that deny their personal worth and truth (worst pole). When both poles exist in a system, the client can also feel pushed and pulled between both of those poles and not see another option. In the third phase of the perspective shift technique, the psychotherapist will invite the client to summarize their LWS in order to begin the process of deepening their understanding of self. Once a deeper understanding of self is set in motion, the psychotherapist can introduce a third pole (mental-emotional space) where observation and further understanding of self can continue outside of the LWS both in and out of session.

Ms. Green: Is it okay if we summarize the work that has been done so far?

Henrietta: Yeah, I have been thinking about that. How do we do that?

Ms. Green: Let's take another look at the paper with the poles and the key points you wrote down about your story (LWS).

Henrietta: Okay.

Ms. Green: When you are ready, review the things you've written (you can talk aloud or to yourself) and give me a summary of what you have been trying to do to survive between the two poles represented on the paper.

Henrietta: Yeah, I got it. (reads and thinks for a few minutes) On the one side, I can't be me at all. That is the worst I feel. I can't show up in the world as me and I won't let myself feel my inherent values because if I let myself embrace that feeling—I could be shunned by my family.

Ms. Green: (nods to show she is listening)

Henrietta: One the other side, the better side. When I accept the conditions in the family and in my relationship with my boyfriend (i.e., heteronormative values), I get acceptance in return. I get invited to family events and told that I matter, and I have a relationship that is allowed. I get to belong, but it is a partial version of me that belongs. I have to pretend that the whole me is less important than the parts of me they prefer.

Ms. Green: ... and as I understand your story and what it has felt like to be stuck between those two different places—it is limiting for you. You don't get to feel whole or worthy in either place.

Henrietta: Yeah, and I thought it was all my fault. That I'm wrong or that I can't do it right.

Ms. Green: Could anyone do it more easily?

Henrietta: (laughs) Oh! Ha! Who would want to do it? It's a crap life.

Ms. Green: It's crappy to be stuck between those poles.

Henrietta: It's the crappiest and suckiest! That's what the poles should be named.

Ms. Green: Have you ever considered that there is a third option?

Henrietta: (raised their eyebrows in curiosity) I didn't even know there were two, so, no.

Ms. Green: Is this an okay place for me to introduce what the third position is?

Henrietta: Sure.

Initiating Perspective Shift Technique Phase 3: Understanding

- The psychotherapist will proceed to describe the existence of a third pole that represents the client's ability to observe themselves without judgment and also experience their original state of BSW. The client can practice moving into the third position to look at the other two poles more objectively. This perspective-taking position can be entered purposefully in session and by the client on their own in order to pause the worth-denying memories/pattern. Once the client enters the third position, they can examine the contents of their LWS in each pole without joining the story-line. Ms. Green invited Henrietta to review the map they co-created in session. This summary or review of contents provides an opportunity for the client to ease into the third pole/position as a perspective-taking exercise. Henrietta was able to take the third position during the session; they looked at the two LWS poles and expressed how they felt. They commented on the price they have paid to live stuck between two poles and what it feels like to be pushed and pulled by their family system's abusive injunctions in one pole, and the conditions of worth in the other.

- In subsequent sessions, the psychotherapist will request that the client return to the map to discuss aspects of their LWS that have caused them to feel stuck. The psychotherapist will remind the client that they have not lost their self-worth; the LWS is a story written about being in a system that lost its worth-based frame of reference, which in some cases occurred generations ago. Consequently, the members of the system may not have felt a tether to their BSW or may not have known how to validate it consistently. Ms. Green will invite Henrietta to resume the third position in future sessions so that they can practice being out of the cycle they have been stuck in. The sessions where the third position is taken are focused on the present moment and how being conscious of having BSW and being worthy can be a common practice.

- As the client begins to feel capable of considering a third pole that will allow them to shift their focus away from the turmoil of worth-denying patterns, the psychotherapist will explain that the third position (pole) existed before the other two poles were learned. In other words, the ability to observe oneself without judgment (i.e., the third position) is akin to an original and unconditioned state of mind that exists at the beginning of life. In support of this notion, Sullivan et al. (2011) reminded us that the ability to observe surroundings and interactions and experience worth as a human being is experienced in the first few years of life. Henrietta was able to write out the contents of their LWS on a piece of paper and place the worst parts of the story and the better parts of the story under the corresponding pole. The successful completion of this exercise means that Henrietta has taken the third position. They can practice shifting into the third position by choosing to observe the patterns, behaviors, and memories that have contributed to denying their BSW. Henrietta hoped it would be helpful to set a timer to see if they could shift into the third position where BSW awaits to be felt and "hang there" for ten minutes. Ms. Green agreed that shifting to the third position and "hanging there" would be a good way to develop a worth-conscious practice. The psychotherapist can offer the idea that practicing the shift in perspective technique helps to disrupt the habitual patterns that are involved in denying BSW. To help the client cultivate this third position where BSW can be affirmed, the psychotherapist can devote a session whereby the client is able to hold themselves in that position.

Session 9: A Mindfulness Technique to Internalize the Third Position

Ms. Green: Think of your mind as a stage.

Henrietta: (closes eyes) Okay.

Ms. Green: Think of all of your thoughts as actors moving on and off that stage.

Henrietta: Woah! That's a lot of action going on.

Ms. Green: Think of your BSW as being center stage. If you have a word you prefer that always helps you feel worthy you can put that word there. Can you see it on the stage just being there?

Henrietta: (nods) I see the words, my worth.

Ms. Green: Watch your worth stay at the center of the stage no matter what all the other actors are doing. Let the thoughts act out whatever scene they are in on the stage and your BSW is unmoved by the action.

Henrietta: Can I put a spotlight on it?

Ms. Green: Sure. Now, what word or phrase can you say that helps keep your sense of worthiness (BSW) solid on the stage of your mind?

Henrietta: I don't know.

Ms. Green: What makes you feel worthy? It can be a memory or a dream of the future.

Henrietta: Like, that I'm good. That I'm kind. Something like that?

Ms. Green: Those are helpful ideas. What words or phrase, when you hear it or think about it, helps you feel worthy as a person?

Henrietta: Oh, I know! That I'm enough. That I'm enough, just as I am.

Ms. Green:　What happens to your worth as you see it on the stage of your mind when you say that phrase to yourself?

Henrietta:　Oh, it's me now. It's me standing there and I am younger.

Ms. Green:　That seems like a powerful phrase for you.

Henrietta:　Is that normal?

Ms. Green:　There isn't a "normal" in this situation, per se. Different phrases work for different clients. We are looking for what affirms your self-worth, when you say it.

Continuation of Phase 3: Initiating Mindfulness

- The psychotherapist can point to the third pole drawn on the paper that they have been referring to during the Understanding phase and say, "This space exists for you to be you." The client is then invited to label the space with a more personalized title such as, me, my worth space, BSW, just being, I'm enough here, okay-ness, and so forth.

- The psychotherapist will let the client sit with this new image on their mental stage for a few moments. They will then explain that the client can occupy the third position space and open up their mental stage to make room for their BSW (i.e., seeing themselves as enough as Henrietta did) on a daily basis. The client is encouraged to allow their BSW or the version of themselves they see as worthy to stay center stage while remaining aware of all the other hundreds of thoughts that move around the stage.

- If the client returns to session reporting a new offense from a family member, the story about the new worth-denying experience can be shared in session. Once the client has expressed their emotions and concerns surrounding the new incident, they can plot the new event on the map. Doing so, will allow the client to once again create a safe space away from the efforts of others who continue to add content to their LWS. Also, the psychotherapist can help the client understand that their LWS is not real; it is not based on their reality as a worthy human being. It seemed real because it was repeated. However, a story can be repeated over and over like *Jack and the Beanstalk* and yet still not become the truth.

Developing Client Worth-Consciousness

To recap the process, the perspective shift technique starts at the point of listening for the possibility of a LWS and concludes with the development of a basic worth-conscious skill set. Once a LWS has been recognized, the client and psychotherapist learn about the contents of that story and how severe the "stuckness" is for the client within their particular worth-denying narrative. The sessions proceed into learning about the LWS (phase two) until the client feels satisfied with the initial mapping of the contents and separates them into the two poles. One pole reflects the worst position in the family system, which is alienation from truth and worth. The second pole is a slightly better position, but is still not healthy since it involves conditions. The sessions continue into phase three (i.e., understanding) with a summary of the aspects of the client's story and how the client has been denied a consistent experience of their self-worth that allows new understanding of an old pattern. The understanding phase can last for several sessions, or be revisited in any future session where the client wants assistance moving away from the pattern of denied or conditional worth and toward building a worth-affirming pattern.

Once the client is able to shift into a third position (third pole) where they can feel safe to observe self and situations from a perspective of being worthy, a worth-conscious mindset is further developed and the client can be introduced to phase four (worth-conscious), which is the last phase of the perspective shift technique.

Worth-Conscious Skill Building

Ms. Green spent some of the time in previous sessions teaching Henrietta about the four pillars of self-worth and the building blocks that make affirming self-worth easier. Ms. Green also shared worth-affirming building blocks with Henrietta to increase self-awareness and self-respect in any session where those blocks were needed. When Henrietta asked for help with a specific thought or situation that denied their worth, Ms. Green invited Henrietta to show which blocks they would have liked to have used in the situation. This was to see if Henrietta already owned some worth-affirming building blocks but did not yet know when to use them. Ms. Green shared worth-affirming building blocks that were new to Henrietta but also checked with them about how likely they were to use those new blocks in their daily life. Ms. Green listened to Henrietta and looked for evidence of the experience of self-esteem and self-confidence, even if they were conditional, to help Henrietta realize that they have some of those building blocks, but the blocks were not grounded in BSW. Lastly, the instruction given on using worth-affirming building blocks included both new and old information that Henrietta had shared or learned in previous sessions where they gained self-awareness, self-respect, self-esteem, or self-confidence grounded in their BSW and that honored their truth and worth congruently.

Tenth Session: Client Learns the Conscious Moment Technique

Henrietta: I have been using the mindfulness technique. I can see the stage in my mind, and I put my self-worth center stage. I have noticed that breathing in slowly while repeating that I'm enough really helps me stay focused on that experience. I see how being mindful uses all of the building blocks in one experience.

Ms. Green: How so?

Henrietta: Well, I'm becoming more aware of my worth, focusing on it is self-respecting, I like how it feels so that helps my self-esteem, and each time I get a little better at it my confidence goes up. I don't know why the breathing helps, but it does.

Ms. Green: Adding breathwork does help with mindfulness. I recommend a five- or six-count breath, if that length of inhale and exhale is comfortable for you. You can also make the word or phrase you are using fill up the whole breath and then repeat it mentally with each inhale and each exhale. It is a little easier to pair the breath with the phrase and keep track of both at the same time.

Henrietta: Can we try that at the end of the session today?

Ms. Green: Yes, I will walk you through how to pair your breathing with the phrase you are using to get into and remain in the third position.

Henrietta: Okay. Now I want to tell you about a new problem that happened at work, that made me feel unworthy and caught me off guard.

Ms. Green: Okay.

Henrietta: One of my colleagues blurted out, What's your deal?! We were in the breakroom, and I was scrolling on my phone, and she just bluntly asked me some pointed questions. I think she likes me and was trying to discover more about me. I wanted to tell her the truth, but I froze.

Ms. Green: Do you have an idea of what you wished you would have said?

Henrietta: I wish I could say, my deal is being Bi, what's your deal? I would like to get to know her better, but I also have a boyfriend that doesn't know I feel this way, so maybe I have to tell him first.

Ms. Green: I can't tell you what is the right order for making that disclosure. I can help you learn a decision-making model about staying conscious of your self-worth while making decisions. It's called the conscious moment technique and it provides a visual of where we shift away from our worth or towards it. May I show it to you?

Henrietta: Yeah.

Ms. Green: (pulled the conscious moment technique chart from her file cabinet) This is the diagram of how to process any life event through a worth-conscious lens. In your situation, you may not have had the time to do this right then, but we can always use the model in session anytime a new event seems to add to your lost-worth story. You can also try it on your own, anytime, when you feel skilled using the model.

Henrietta: Okay, so, how do I use it.

Ms. Green: See the M square at the bottom center of the page (**refer back to Figure 8.1 for the conscious moment technique**).

Henrietta: (Nodded)

Ms. Green: That is the point of choosing a worth-affirming direction or a worth-denying direction. In the breakroom, which direction did you want to go (using the model)?

Henrietta: I wanted to be myself and tell my truth to her, but I stopped myself.

Ms. Green: Did any of the conditions, requirements, or rules from your family system enter your mind as a reason to stop?

Henrietta: They did after I came to my senses again. I thought woah, I can't tell her something that my family doesn't know.

Ms. Green: Does one of the rules you have followed sound something like, don't talk about being bisexual?

Henrietta: Well, I can't talk about it, so I don't.

Ms. Green: Let's put that statement on the conscious moment technique chart to see where you go with it.

Henrietta: I already know it takes me left. (puts finger on the chart and drags it to the self-conscious box) If I talk about it to one person, then I might talk about it to people who don't want to hear it. I'm very self-conscious about it.

Ms. Green: Do you want to continue to put the first statement through the model or do you want to switch to this secondary problem?

Henrietta: The first statement, talking about being bisexual. It's the bigger issue.

Ms. Green: Let's put that idea on the conscious moment chart. Would any of the building blocks you already have help you move from not knowing what to do to doing something that affirms your worth? (pulled the building blocks chart from her files; see Figure 8.6)

Henrietta: First, I'm aware that I talk about it with you, in here, with no fear. And I don't hate myself when we talk about it, is that maybe more self-respect too?

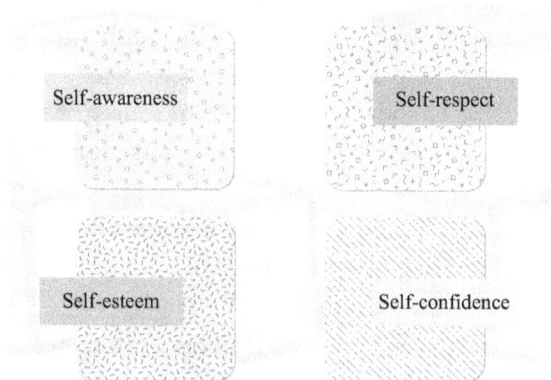

Self-awareness	Self-respect
Self-esteem	Self-confidence

Figure 8.6 Building Blocks.

Ms. Green: Does not hating yourself when you talk about something real for you feel more respectful of your truth?

Henrietta: It does, and that is different for me.

Ms. Green: Does being true to yourself seem like a worth-affirming choice?

Henrietta: It feels like I think I'm enough (their eyes tear up a little).

Initiating Perspective Shift Technique Phase 4: Gaining Worth-Conscious

- The psychotherapist will introduce the conscious moment technique as an additional tool that the client can use in session until they become proficient at using it to shift from the routinized disbelief in their self-worth to affirmation of their BSW. The client can take a copy of the conscious moment model home to help with identifying any worth-denying thoughts that shift them back into the old pattern. Henrietta practiced the skill in session by identifying a worth-denying statement that was a big part of their LWS.

- During phases 1 and 2, the psychotherapist has listened to and learned about their client's LWS. During phase 4, the psychotherapist will pay attention to any of the building blocks that the client has already used to help them manage the stuckness they have experienced. When the psychotherapist becomes aware of a building block that can be useful to helping the client affirm their self-worth, they can mention it at that time or take note of it to discuss later. Henrietta was able to identify where some of their worth-affirming building blocks fit during the mindfulness discussion and the conscious moment instruction.

- This phase is a continuation of the practice of internalizing self-worth and visualizing it by using the mind-is-a-stage exercise. The client can elect to initiate or end a session with the mindfulness exercise (phase 3) as a way to remember how to move into the third position. At the end of a session during phase 4, Henrietta asked to include the mindfulness technique that they learned in phase 3. Ms. Green saw the benefit of assisting Henrietta in returning to the mind as a stage technique so that they could reinforce and internalize a perspective shift that affirms their BSW.

The psychotherapist will bring the client's attention to the two distinctly different moves with different outcomes. The client can choose a move toward denying self-worth (i.e., self-conscious outcome), or they can move toward affirming their self-worth with the help of self-affirming building blocks (i.e., worth-conscious outcome). As related to Henrietta, Ms. Green was able to request that Henrietta explore whether being their true self was a worth affirming choice.

The complete perspective shift process (phases 1–4) may require more sessions in each phase per the client's needs than we have demonstrated in this chapter. Each psychotherapist who uses the perspective shift technique can determine client readiness, pace during phase, and length of each phase based on their knowledge of the client they are working with. The phases as therapeutic processes provide an opportunity for the psychotherapist to recognize any building blocks the client already possesses and uses. Even the client's conditional building blocks (e.g., do not identify as bisexual as a sign of parental respect in the case of Henrietta) can be named as their best effort of accessing the only building blocks that were allowed in their family system. In the fourth and final phase, the psychotherapist and client review the building blocks that the client is proficient at using. Together, they also discuss what is useful or worth affirming about those blocks, including which ones, if any, can be salvaged to serve the client's self-worth needs.

Affirming Building Blocks Used in the Pillars of Self-Worth

A client does not have to suffer the adverse effects of a LWS in order to benefit from learning worth-affirming processes. In other words, learning to affirm one's worth is a critical step toward bolstering wellness, which should be reinforced with or without the experience of a LWS. The client may discover that they have and use building blocks for three of the four pillars of self-worth and need help gathering blocks specific to their one unfinished pillar. Building blocks are the thoughts, words, and actions in a moment that support BSW and help align the client to their truth. When a lack of awareness about one's worth and truth is present, it is possible that the other three pillars of worth (i.e., self-respect, self-esteem, and self-confidence) are not fully built. When the self-awareness pillar is built, it is inaugural to recognize one's truth and worth, which makes building the three remaining worth-based pillars possible.

Yet another consideration for learning worth-affirming processes in the absence of a LWS is when a client has had the experience of one caregiver who helped them build their pillars on a foundation of BSW and another caregiver who influenced them to build on conditional worth in pursuit of a counterfeit. In this example, the client has two separate buildings they have been constructing and they may be familiar with using building blocks that support worth in some ways but deny it in others. This client may have had to conform to intrusive injunctions which can include following a set of acquired family values that are also reinforced by the larger community, making the client conditionally acceptable to family and the larger community. This limited acceptability makes it more difficult to discern one's truth from the required conditions.

The WCT model can be taught as a way for clients to think about aligning their thoughts and actions to their truth and worth. A WCT frame of reference encourages clients to work on building the pillar(s) that they care to build. When a psychotherapist knows what self-worth pillar the client wants help using, together, they can focus on where, when, and how to use the blocks (i.e., moments that are always worth affirming for the client) that belong in that pillar more often. Further in this chapter, we provide three dialogues of client and psychotherapist dialogue exchange in which the client is using building blocks within specific pillars of self-worth and the psychotherapist affirms the client's actions. In these dialogues, a condition exists in the family system, thereby resulting in conditional worth for the client (see Dialogues 1 and 3) or the client has been unsuccessful with using the identifiable building block as a worth-affirming action either with themselves or in their interactions with others (see Dialogue 2). In each dialogue, the adult client is provided an opportunity in session to learn to use the worth-affirming building blocks. There are many iterations of the utility of the WCT model for different clients who have differing degrees of incongruency between worth and truth, or who have truth and conditional worth with some worth-affirming blocks in use on a consistent basis. These clients do not have a LWS that is debilitating, but they have felt the lack of recognition of their worth often enough that reinforcing worth-affirming processes are beneficial.

Worth-Affirming Moments

Affirming self-worth at its simplest level is saying yes to it. In psychotherapy, even though the psychotherapist is observing the client's state of denied or affirmed self-worth they are also participating in affirming (saying yes to) their client's self-worth as a birthright. Passive affirmation of the client's worth by the psychotherapist involves using some basic blocks from the four pillars of self-worth. For example, the psychotherapist listens for what causes the client to shift out of feeling worthy, respects the client no matter which state they are experiencing (i.e., denied or conditional), esteems the client as worth the time it takes to observe and assess for their degree of denied self-worth, and trusts that the client is competent to tell their life story to the best of their ability. In summary, passive affirmation of client BSW is simply holding space for the client in a way that allows whatever amount of worthiness they experience to surface and be witnessed.

The psychotherapist can move from passive observer into a more active affirmation of client worth when the psychotherapist notices the client using any of the building blocks from their own four pillars of self-worth during a session. For example, the client is aware of something true about them that has not been affirmed because it is not valued in the family system. Sometimes parents are unaware and therefore cannot model awareness of a personal truth the child experiences. Other times, parents are aware of an experience the child is having and devalue it as wrong, weird, or unnecessary to achieving the goals the family has set. Therefore, self-awareness of the truth is not fostered, and the child may be left to guess about the worth of that truth. Worth-affirming psychotherapy makes room for personal truth. In any session where a client begins to speak about a true experience that was not allowed or valued, the psychotherapist stays open and aware of the timing that is preferred by the client in sharing about the invalidation of their truth by the outside world. The psychotherapist may use head nods, a smile, or words that signify the valuing of the building blocks (i.e., thoughts/words/actions) that the client uses in the story about their everyday life. The client can be redirected toward considering using any building blocks that affirm their self-worth and away from using building blocks that have been employed in building imitation pillars that affirm conditional worth or deny their worth. An even more actively affirming stance can be used by the psychotherapist when the client is interested in using worth-consciousness as a frame of reference. In other words, holding worth-consciousness as a frame of reference reminds the client to unapologetically practice their truth and worth throughout their lifetime. The following dialogue, provided in Dialogue 1, represents the client's self-awareness of their lived truth since leaving home. While in session, the client depicted in Dialogue 1 shared the awareness they developed in adulthood that was not possible in childhood because the family system could not make room for them to think outside the set of valued norms already established.

Dialogue 1. Self-awareness Building Block is in Use and Affirmed in Session

Client: So, growing up in my family I was encouraged to talk more and be more social. My mother would call friends for me and put me on the phone to confirm with friends that I would leave the house to meet up with them that day. I was an introvert in a family full of extroverts and they didn't get me.

Psychotherapist: (reflecting sentiment) You were a lone introvert?

Client: I had never heard of the idea of being introverted. The terms introvert or extrovert were never used. Being introverted was a bad thing in my family, that behavior meant I was broken.

Psychotherapist: (affirming awareness) You seem more aware of being introverted now.

If the client responds that they have more awareness, the psychotherapist can summarize the idea of introversion being misunderstood as a type of brokenness and invite the client to assess for building blocks they already have, such as looking for the presence of self-respect for self as an introvert.

Psychotherapist: Living true to your introversion today, do you respect that about yourself?

Client:	Yes, it feels normal. I can't not be this way.
Psychotherapist:	Do you think your family was aware of introversion as a possibility?
Client:	No, they didn't know how hard I tried to be like them. I didn't understand that none of them were trying like I was; they were just being them.
Psychotherapist:	Does the awareness and respect you have for yourself as an introvert, now, help you feel true to yourself even when you are with family who don't understand that about you?
Client:	They don't get it, but they don't disbelieve me anymore.

Each pillar of worth gives the psychotherapist a range of responses from the clients' point of view. They can explore which blocks the client may already have and which ones the client has used to build each pillar of self-worth that mirrors their true experience. The psychotherapist's questions and/or responses to the client can be tailored to fit the style of expression that the psychotherapist prefers as long as their questions and responses affirm the truth the client is experiencing with the building blocks the client is comfortable using.

Examples of Questions from each Pillar of Self-Worth that the Psychotherapist Might Find Useful:

Self-awareness affirming
What are you aware of?
Did you become more aware?
Has your awareness continued to increase?
Was awareness lacking at the time?

Self-respect affirming
Is that an increase in self-respect?
Do you respect that about yourself?
Did you feel disrespected then?

Self-esteem affirming
What do you like about that?
Was that easier to like than before?
Did positive feelings about yourself increase?

You like that about your friend (cousin/partner)?

<u>Self-confidence affirming</u>

Do you trust that about yourself?

Did you feel more capable?

You showed up for yourself?

Did you pretend it didn't bother you?

The closed questions listed above are provided to solicit a 'yes' or 'no' response from the client to a specific piece of information in their life story. Open questions are also listed and used to help the client explore their story and learn how their pattern of conditional or denied self-worth strays into new relationships at work, with neighbors, and with acquaintances in their community. Affirming the building blocks that are in use and that help the client affirm both their lived truth and their BSW is directive in the sense that the therapist is choosing the direction of the process in that moment. Jay Hayley (1976) suggested that a psychotherapist give directives when assuming the task of initiating what happens in the session. He offered the possibility of overtly telling a client to stop doing something. We are suggesting a gentler approach, which includes directing the client toward worth-affirming building blocks as an agreed-upon treatment goal for one or more sessions. Instead of telling the client to stop something, the psychotherapist can invite the client to practice thoughts, words, or actions that affirm their worth (reinforcing the pillars) as they rewrite their life story.

Hayley (1976) also indicated that direction from a psychotherapist be precise, which involves giving clear instructions. The client can be introduced to the idea of self-worth as a theme in psychotherapy; when the client agrees to explore how self-worth has been missing from their personal narrative, they can also be introduced to WCT concepts. When the client shares specific life events, the psychotherapist informs the client that they are listening for when and where certain worth-affirming building blocks have been used to affirm the client's self-worth or not. Throughout the therapeutic process, the client is reminded to indicate whether they agree with the psychotherapist's observations or not. The client is respected as the expert in their life experiences and holds the knowledge that is needed to become worth-conscious of their lived truth.

If a therapeutic observation is confirmed by the client as being helpful, the client can keep the information to use for further inspection. The client is supported in gaining understanding about when and where self-worth-affirming building blocks help them practice being worthy.

Cleaning Up Communication

Communication tells us about the world. The signals we feel inside our body are communicated to that world, making them aware of our internal experience. What the outside world communicates back to us can complicate our ability to understand how communicating the truth is beneficial in the system. Messages can be misheard, misunderstood, or misinterpreted by caregivers. Without the benefit of clarification, mixed messages can become the components in building blocks that children learn to use that promote mind or power games, instead of accuracy of understanding. The simplicity of two bits of communication, such as an uncomplicated yes or no, was introduced by physicist John Wheeler (1989) as something so basic in physics that it is foundational in our participatory universe. Wheeler shared the importance of information being simplified by a yes-no process. Wheeler believed that everything is made up of bits, which are binary yes-or-no pieces of information that matter. Borrowing the usefulness of a yes-no process uncomplicates our understanding of how self-worth is denied or affirmed. In the history of each client, there may be a pattern of denied self-worth that showed up as rejections (i.e., a no response) to their lived experience in the form of injunctions, requirements, and objections to what was true for the client in childhood. A pattern of conditional self-worth can include verbal or nonverbal acceptance (i.e., a yes but response) to the client's worth in childhood that had a qualifying "only if" condition attached to it.

Similarly, Hayley (1976) noted that the precision of communication can be reduced to each statement having only one referent, which allows for one signal and one response (such as a yes or no). In this case, each message or statement is about one thing and cannot be about any other thing, which allows for the reduction of uncertainty. In his chapter on Information Theory, Griffin (1994) referenced Shannon and Weaver's model of communication (1949), which suggested that eliminating uncertainty reduces entropy (i.e., a degree of disorder). When entropy is reduced, certainty is increased, and communication is less complicated. According to Shannon and Weaver (as cited in Griffin, 1994), clear ways of communicating can cut entropy in half. Shannon and Weaver provided an example of uncluttered communication in action, which we have modified and shared below:

> Imagine making a phone call where you are responding to a friend who heard a rumor about you having a fling with a co-worker. The friend sent a text asking about the rumor and ended with this request: Call me and just say "yes", it's true, or "no" it's not—no more. The clear communication demanding one of two responses meant the phone conversation would not take as long. The request also dropped the friend's uncertainty to fifty percent as there was only two bits of information required.

Even with reducing the response options to yes or no, a truth can be contradicted accidentally or purposefully. When the contradiction is accidental, like a parent saying you can't be hungry to a child who is hungry because she ran the equivalent of two miles playing in the backyard, the child may have recourse to counter their parent's misinterpretation and have their truth heard. When the contradiction to the child's truth is purposeful because the parent does not care if the child is hungry, the child can try to be heard, but there may be a punishment for correcting the contradicting message. This is a two-knot problem because the child's internal "Yes" to feeling hungry is countered with a parental, "No, you are not!" A yes response that is paired with a no causes a knot (see Figure 8.7). This is the first knot in this illustration because the parent is saying no to the child's truth (i.e., hunger), and this is followed by the child trying to reassert their truth, "But I am", which is met with another parental counter, "Don't say another word. You are not eating right now." This would be the second knot because it is a second counter to the truth that the child

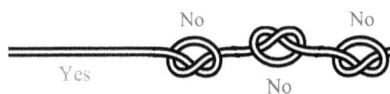

Figure 8.7 The Yes and No Knot.

is experiencing. A triple knot would occur if the parent made an assertion about the child that was not true for them like, "You're lying." This third knot hits the child's worth more deeply because it speaks to the parent's denial of the child's truth telling.

When we simplify things down to a yes response that affirms self-worth and a no that denies self-worth, we can see the mess of mixed messages more clearly. The client, as an adult, may be trying to unravel the mix of external counters to their original signals about their truth. The inaccurate responses from parents, and others, which negate an experienced truth can show up in psychotherapy as a tangle of yes and no knots that are familiar and have denied the client's worth and disregarded their truth. The original yes (to who I am and what I am experiencing) that the child received about being hungry, tired, joyful, or accurate about their truth validates not only their experience but their ability to trust that their experience matters. Let us remember that a signal of hunger is true for the child but if a denial of hunger is communicated by a parent, the child receives a confusing no, which counters their true yes. This can send a message to the child that parental power is more important than knowing what is real—demanding denial of truth and its worth in the moment.

The conflict of interest for the child when a no (denial) response is given to their yes (affirming) is not always a known phenomenon in the family system. The parents may unknowingly move against a child's lived truth, as noted with the introvert in a family of extroverts described in Dialogue 1. A move against the child's truth can increase entropy for the child who is living with an internal yes, and who would benefit from an external yes from the people they are trusting to be responsible observers/models for them. Kazdin (1994) offered the notion that people learn behaviors/activities without ever being reinforced for performing them. Observational learning (i.e., modeling) occurs when an individual, such as a child, observes the model engaging in a behavior and imitates it. This may account for how families pass down rules that dictate and ignore the BSW of certain members of the family. A parent who perpetually asserts their set of values as the only way to live, over honoring their child's inherent values, may mean well but their actions deny their child's truth. Requiring the child's allegiance to a set of values that is counter to their truth renders the child conditionally worthy and/or complicit in denying what is true for them.

The knot diagram shows how more complicated the knot becomes when there are countering moves (i.e., additional no responses) by parents to a child's insistence that their yes is real. When a parental "no" was given to counter the child's internally helpful yes, the child may try again to restate the truth of their yes. The child who persisted, and was allowed to resist the parents' counter move, may have strengthened their held truth and more easily kept living true to their internal yes. If resistance was futile in the family system, due to exigencies, the internal yes of the child may have been replaced with a parent's preferred no, and the client in psychotherapy, having accepted that alternative to their reality, may not know where to begin to unravel the knot.

To clean up communication in psychotherapy the client may be unaware of how many knots they have in their thinking about themselves, and where their truth and worth have become incongruent. The client may have knotted thinking that affects just one pillar of self-worth (e.g., self-respect) more than others, but they could also have knotted thinking that effects more than one pillar of worth. The WCT-trained psychotherapist will listen for a client's lived truth (affirming) while holding space for the client to feel worthy (affirming). The psychotherapist is listening for truth that has been countered and worth that has been rerouted in the service of a counterfeit through conditions. Knot-free or clean communication about truth and worth is a client story that resembles this: "Growing up, I had a foundation of worth available in my family system that supported my self-discovery. The many truths I learned about myself over the years were grounded in being worthy of knowing and being me all along the way." Honoring individual worth without obstructing personal truth is one of the goals with clients in session.

In WCT, we look at a reduction in confusion that simple yes/no responses can provide as vital to making individual truth/worth accessible. This may reduce the complications of familial/observer bias which has become acceptable to the client. Parents, as the original observers, have a set of values that can be acquired by the children in the family (for good or ill), but that set of values may move against one or more of the child's inherent values. This sets up a contradiction of communication that can complicate the sense of self. When the child has an internal yes to something personally experienced as true for them, but that same experience is responded to with a no from the parents, the child has to either choose their truth (i.e., something that can be inherently valued as real for them) or the acceptable alternative in that family system, which inadvertently requires the child to tell themselves no. Once the child accepts a counter (i.e., no) as the required response to the parents, they become complicit to counter moves displacing their honest yes. As previously noted, an internal yes that is met with an external no that must be accepted as superior to the honest yes, is the first twist in the knot. The knot will have more twists for clients who are burdened with a LWS. These clients have experienced an internal yes that was met with at least two external no responses—a no response to their experience and a second no to the sharing of that experience.

The more complicated a knot of mixed messages becomes, the more it can resemble the six characteristics of the double-bind predicament outlined by Nichols and Schwartz (1998). First, communication involves two or more people who have an important emotional relationship with one of them holding positional power, such as a parent. Second, the pattern of communication is repeated. Third, the communication involves a primary negative injunction (i.e., *Do not do so and so, or I will punish you*, or *If you do not do so and so, I will punish you*) from the person with positional power or a command not to do something on threat of punishment. Fourth, the communication also involves a second abstract requirement with a threat of punishment that contradicts the first command; thereby, confusing the receiver. Fifth, a third command both demands a response and prevents escape, effectively binding the recipient into a no-win situation. Sixth, the recipient is conditioned to participate through repetition of the steps until they become complicit in the process making the enactment of all six steps of the pattern unnecessary to keep the child bound/stuck (i.e., confused and disempowered). In other words, once the recipient is groomed, it only takes a glance/stare from the person who holds the positional power to move the recipient into submission. To illustrate the double-bind communication between a parent and their child we offer the following example:

A parent informs their child that in this family we express our feelings openly and honestly and requests the same of the child. When the child hears the command and proceeds to share their feelings, the parent simultaneously exhibits anger and/or disapproval. Consequently, the child may feel as though they are being commanded to communicate and at the same time punished for doing so. The parent is then critical of the child's lack of sharing. To put it another way, both the child's attempt to talk and their lack of sharing are punished; hence, the double-bind (i.e., no-win predicament). The meaning of communication becomes unclear for the child and in the future, they may display hesitancy with expressing their feelings despite being encouraged to be open.

Whereas double-bind messaging creates turmoil because truth and worth are denied, a wellness-focused alternative style of communication involves an affirming transaction of internal to external communication where communication is uncomplicated by counter moves.

Internal to External Communication

The simplest transaction of internal to external communication using an example of hunger as a basic life need involves four steps. The first step is that the stomach sends a signal to the brain that hunger exists. When this communication process is clean, the brain registers the signal as a 'yes' this is true. The second step is that the original signal is conveyed outwardly/externally by vocalizing hunger as a life need. If the caregiver is present and responds to the need, that interaction becomes the second 'yes'. In the third step, when the need is fulfilled, the wiring of the brain and the body connection is strengthened, and the hunger signal will be repeated. When this need is repeated and the caregiver consistently responds to the signal as true, the child comes to learn that what is true to them is valued, which is the third 'yes' in this chain of communication. In step four, when physiological needs are met consistently, there is a relational connection that is established, and this is where self-worth is introduced. The brain recognizes that this exchange (i.e., relational connection) matters, which is the fourth 'yes' and also the origin of worth consciousness. These four steps are repeated with every life need and with every relational exchange

Table 8.1 An Affirming Chain of Communication

Signals	Responses
1. Original hunger signal	Brain of child recognizes the signal with a yes, it's true (yes #1).
2. Signal is communicated	Caregiver responds to signal and feeds (yes #2)
3. Signal is working	Caregiver cares about the signal's truth (yes #3).
4. My signals matter	Brain of child recognizes that this exchange matters (yes #4).

where self-worth is affirmed. See Table 8.1 for signals and responses that create an affirming chain of communication.

Signals and Responses

Critical to our work with clients is understanding how their childhood and adult signals have been communicated and met. An internal and physical signal, such as hunger, can become trusted by the child because it tells the truth about the child's physical state. In addition, when the exhibited need (i.e., hunger) is met with food by a caregiver, the child learns to trust that they are worth caring for. An external yes by the caregiver to the internal yes of the child's physical state (i.e., my hunger is real) creates a congruency that can be trusted. Both physical and emotional signals are important. Physical signals (i.e., basic life needs) are more cut and dried in that they support life and when not met the child will not survive. Emotional signals must also be understood and met. With mental and/or emotional needs, differences in personality may be at play. The emergence of differences in temperament (i.e., a precursor to personality) can occur as young as age three (McAdams & Olson, 2010). Although longitudinal data are relatively scarce, some findings show a connection between temperament and personality characteristics. More specifically, the landmark longitudinal study of a thousand children born in Dunedin, New Zealand documented statistically significant associations between age 3 temperaments and personality traits by age 26 (Caspi et al. 2003). To further clarify, some babies cry at sounds that make other babies laugh. Which baby is displaying the correct response? Both babies are likely telling the truth about something inside of them. One baby's truth is illustrated in the example below.

A baby started to cry when his mother opened a hard candy that was wrapped in a noisy piece of plastic. The mother laughed at the baby's response because there was nothing to be afraid of; she had not expected the baby to cry when he heard the plastic twisted away from the candy. The baby heard an unfamiliar sound that alerted something in his mind which was followed by a cry of discomfort. The mother laughed because her experience was different, her laugh was an external 'no' to the baby's internal 'yes' of fearing the noise. In this case, the incongruency between internal experience of the child and the life experience of the parent was followed by the mother attending to the child's discomfort, by picking him up and speaking softly. This comforting behavior provided a 'yes' to the truth the child seemed to experience (fear), even though the mother did not share the appraisal of the experience. The baby being worth the comfort even though the cause of the fear was not shared may have been related to the low level of awareness of a baby at that age. There was an external signal (something fearful) that caused an internal alert, an external 'no' (not fearful) from mom, but with an affirming worth move (i.e., nonverbal yes) that communicated you feel afraid so I will comfort you even though you are not in danger.

As psychotherapists, when we recognize our clients' signals as simple yes or no responses to their lived truth, we can help them to easily discern what has influenced them away from their truth and toward conditional or denied worth in their family system. The psychotherapist assumes an important role in helping clients to untangle any mental and/or emotional knots that keep them confused about their truth, their internal signals, and remaining worthy. In essence, the psychotherapist listens for the denial of truth or worth in the story the client shares. In WCT, we regard the client's telling of their life story as their journey toward uncovering their truth and trusting that, when communicated, their truth matters. Certainly, there is benefit when one's lived truth and individual worth comingled early in their child development; however, that may not be the case for many clients who seek psychotherapy. In WCT, truth about self is experienced throughout the developmental phases. The young child from birth to age 12 is beginning to experience their signals and understand how their signals help them learn what is true for them. They are learning about the signals that happen in their body and mind and if they are valued by others. Over time, the practice of experiencing personal truth plus being worthy throughout those experiences combine to provide a life of realized self-worth. Signals that are universally known (e.g., hunger, fear) and also specific to the individual (e.g., personality characteristics), occur over time and become wired (i.e., the communication becomes repeated or extinguished) by responses that are affirmed or denied.

Internal signals are not the only information coming into the brain. The five senses are taking in information through visual, auditory, tactile, gustatory, and olfactory paths. This information signals to the brain what exists in the outer world. As the client developed, they may have become aware of signals that systems outside the family sent to anyone watching. For example, commercials on television can signal to a female client that if she looks good in the clothing a particular merchant is selling, she will be desired. This signal is not rooted in the client's known truth and may not support their worth, but the client can agree with the commercial and that agreement can turn into a personally held requirement that moves against her sense of self (i.e., her truth and worth).

The following client, presented in Dialogue 2, had acquired a value from watching television commercial ads that unknowingly infringed on her self-esteem. The acquired value of having a smaller body size as reflected in those ads contributed to her devaluing herself as a desired romantic partner. She did not esteem herself as a desirable woman after accepting *the world* (larger community value) view of her body.

Dialogue 2: Self-esteem Building Blocks are not Worth-Based but Rather World-Based

Client:	I don't initiate sex with my partner, and I feel bad because I love them.
Psychotherapist:	We have discussed this issue in the past. Is there something you need me to know about this today?
Client:	Yes, I think it's because I have no self-esteem.

Psychotherapist:	How so?
Client:	I don't want them to see me naked, because I have gained fifty pounds since we met.
Psychotherapist:	So, does weight affect your self-esteem?
Client:	I am not desirable anymore. So, that makes me feel bad about myself.
Psychotherapist:	Has your partner mentioned to you that you aren't desirable?
Client:	No, they are totally into me. I don't know why.
Psychotherapist:	You don't know why someone desires you?
Client:	Yeah, I wouldn't have sex with me.
Psychotherapist:	Is there a requirement for you to engage?
Client:	Yeah (laughs), skinny people are sexy! I'm not that, at all.
Psychotherapist:	(pauses) You're saying you don't fit a certain definition of sexy. Do the two of you share a definition of desirability?
Client:	No, but it was easier when I felt sexy.
Psychotherapist:	It was easier when you fit the definition of sexy in your mind.
Client:	Yes, the definition the world says is sexy.
Psychotherapist:	Can we look at the worth-affirming building blocks you have to see how this statement measures up?
Client:	Sure. I like to be aware; I like to be respectful, I like when I have self-esteem, and I enjoy feeling confident.
Psychotherapist:	I see that you remember the different pillars of self-worth.
Client:	Yes.
Psychotherapist:	When you think about the world's definition of what it means to be sexy, can you be more aware of how you accepted that as part of your story?
Client:	That I have failed at being it.
Psychotherapist:	Can I use that statement and put it into the worst category?
Client:	Yes.

Psychotherapist:	Writing worst outcome on a dry erase board and adding the word failed under it. If that's the worst outcome, what is a better worth-affirming option?
Client:	Ha, ha! If I knew, I wouldn't be having this problem.
Psychotherapist:	What would a worth-based statement about your body sound like?
Client:	That I am not sexy, but that's life?
Psychotherapist:	Do you feel more self-respect when you say that?
Client:	Nope.
Psychotherapist:	Is there a worth-based statement that includes awareness, respect, or esteem?
Client:	I can't think of one.
Psychotherapist:	Would it help to consider how you think about the desirability of your partner?
Client:	My partner deserves my love even though they are imperfect. I never question that!
Psychotherapist:	What are you aware of when you make that statement?
Client:	My partner is worth it and imperfect. I guess I don't think of them as sexy or not sexy.
Psychotherapist:	So, they get loved without the conditions the world has put on you?
Client:	I guess so. I give my partner better than I give myself.
Psychotherapist:	There is good news in that. If you see others as worthy of your love, you have esteem building blocks and are using them; you just haven't added your name to the blocks. Can we try to use them for you, too?
Client:	(sighs) That may take some time to accomplish.
Psychotherapist:	(recognizes resistance) Let's look at the esteem blocks you use that say, my partner has changed over time, and you still like them. What would that sound like if it were written for you?

The client and psychotherapist would use the time left to continue looking at any additional building blocks being used to affirm the worth of the partner but not yet being used to affirm the client's self-worth. This can be limited to one of the pillars of self-worth (such as esteem for...) or the client can be given space to jump around picking up the building blocks they see as helpful in rewriting this part of their story. The conscious moment technique can also be useful to show the client and help her see that what she calls the "world's standard" makes her feel self-conscious, and ultimately denies her own worth.

Signals and Responses in Conflict

In psychotherapy, giving the client permission to be worthy and true to self may be in conflict with the acceptance they receive in their family system. It may also be in conflict with a set of rules that helped them survive in the system where they are still active members. This can set up an internal conflict for the client to resist making worth-affirming choices that could affect their membership in their family system. A client can be comfortable with the conditions required to be accepted by their family and therefore not want to disrupt the status quo. Yet, another client may want to learn about and use worth-affirming building blocks but discover that they cannot enjoy using a new skill with one or more family members because the skill is rebuffed as ridiculous or even offensive. To further clarify, see Dialogue 3, in which a client is feeling distressed in session about an event at work that they cannot tolerate, but the solution involves using self-respecting building blocks that are not allowed at home. The client became uncomfortable thinking about using *forbidden blocks*—their uncomfortableness can be addressed overtly and with the yes/no simplicity employed. The psychotherapist would get permission from the client to use closed questions for this exercise. The client would choose which pillar of self-worth to be directed towards for this exercise.

Dialogue 3: Self-Respect Building Block Hesitancy

Psychotherapist: Can we look at something more specific about this building block that we are starting to practice using in your interactions with others?

Client: Sure. We were working on using the self-respect building block of correcting errors made on the project at work.

Psychotherapist:	Are you able to give me a yes or no response to a few questions about this building block you want to use more often?
Client:	Yes.
Psychotherapist:	Okay, does talking about being more self-respecting feel uncomfortable?
Client:	Yes, but I don't know why.
Psychotherapist:	Okay, does the discomfort happen when you think about being self-respecting at work?
Client:	No, not at all.
Psychotherapist:	Does the discomfort happen when you think about being self-respecting with family (or state the specific way)?
Client:	Yes, with my dad.
Psychotherapist:	Can you use this self-respecting block in here as we work together?
Client:	Yes.
Psychotherapist:	Does that make you more or less comfortable in here?
Client:	Can I say more than yes or no to that?
Psychotherapist:	Of course. Thanks for being aware of the rules of this exercise.
Client:	Yes, I'm uncomfortable but it's because I feel sad. Like… you just let me catch you making an error and correct you without becoming a jerk. I can't do that with my dad. I need to do that at work. I have to catch errors and ask my team to correct them daily.
Psychotherapist:	So, in therapy and at work you get to recognize an error and ask about that error being made by someone and many of the people you do this with can handle that you see something they missed?
Client:	Yes, but I get sick to my stomach like I am doing something that will get me in trouble.
Psychotherapist:	Being respectful and respected is not always allowed?
Client:	If I don't feel respected here or at work, I can say so.
Psychotherapist:	Is it okay with you to practice the self-respecting skill here and at work but not yet use it at home with your dad?

Client: Yes, can I do that? I thought I had to use the building
                 blocks with everyone.
Psychotherapist: It's an interesting idea that you can explore. If you want
                 to be more self-respecting in a specific way and there
                 are already safe people to practice with then practicing
                 with them is an option. Getting familiar with the skill
                 may happen best with safe people.
Client: That sounds easier and less uncomfortable.

The psychotherapist would continue to support the client in identifying
and practice using self-respect building blocks that affirm his worth. As
the client continues to practice self-respect building blocks in safe spaces
and in interactions with others where he feels comfortable, he will be
invited to share his readiness to be more self-respecting in his communication with his father, if he has not already done so.

References

Caspi, A., Harrington, H. L., Milne, B., Amell, J.W., Theodore, R.F., & Moffitt, T. E. (2003). Children's behavioral styles at age 3 are linked to their adult personality traits at age 26. *Journal of Personality, 71*, 495–513.

Ciarrocchi, J., Bailey, A., & Harris, R. (2013). *The weight escape: How to stop dieting and start living*. Melbourne, Victoria: Penguin Books Australia.

Griffin, E. A. (1994). *A first look at communication theory*. (2nd ed.). New York: McGraw-Hill.

Harris, R. (2019). *ACT made simple: An easy-to-read primer on acceptance and commitment therapy*. (2nd ed.). Oakland, CA: New Harbinger Publications.

Hayes, S. C. (2004). Acceptance and commitment therapy, relational frame theory, and the third wave of behavioral and cognitive therapies. *Behavior Therapy, 35*, 639–665. https://doi.org/10.1016/S0005-7894(04)80013-3

Hayes, S. C., Levin, M. E., Plumb-Vilardaga, J., Villatte, J. L., & Pistorello, J. (2013). Acceptance and commitment therapy and contextual behavioral science: Examining the progress of a distinctive model of behavioral and cognitive therapy. *Behavior therapy, 44*(2), 180–198. https://doi.org/10.1016/j.beth.2009.08.002

Hayley, J. (1976). *Problem Solving Therapy: New strategies for effective family therapy*. San Francisco, CA: Jossey-Bass Publishers.

Kazdin, A. E. (1994). *Behavior modification in applied settings*. (5th ed.). Pacific Grove, CA: Brooks/Cole.

Konnikova, M. (2014). *What's lost as handwriting fades*. June 2. New York Times.

McAdams, D. P., & Olson, B. D. (2010). Personality development: Continuity and change over the life course. *Annual Review of Psychology, 61*(1), 517–542.

Nichols, M. P., & Schwartz, R. C. (1998). *Family therapy: Concepts and methods*. (4th ed.).Boston, MA: Allyn & Bacon.

Siegel, Daniel J., (1999). *The developing mind: Toward a neurobiology of interpersonal experience*. New York: Guilford Press.

Sullivan, R., Perry, R., Sloan, A., Kleinhaus, K., & Burtchen, N. (2011). Infant bonding and attachment to caregivers: Insights from basic and clinical science. *Clinics in Perinatology, 38*(4), 643–655. https://doi.org/10.1016/j.clp.2011.08.011

Tangney, J. P., & Dearing, R. L. (2002). *Shame and guilt.* New York, NY, USA: Guilford Press.

Wheeler, J. A. (1989). Information, physics, quantum: the search for links, *Proceedings III of the International Symposium on Foundations of Quantum Mechanics.* Tokyo, 1989, 354–368.

INDEX

Pages in *italics* refer to figures and pages in **bold** refer to tables.

For Product Safety Concerns and Information please contact our EU
representative GPSR@taylorandfrancis.com
Taylor & Francis Verlag GmbH, Kaufingerstraße 24, 80331 München, Germany